MENTAL ILLNESSES AND TREATMENTS

DRUG ADDICTION, TRAUMA, AND MENTAL ILLNESS

INTERPRETATION AND INTERVENTION

MENTAL ILLNESSES AND TREATMENTS

Additional books and e-books in this series can be found on Nova's website under the Series tab.

MENTAL ILLNESSES AND TREATMENTS

DRUG ADDICTION, TRAUMA, AND MENTAL ILLNESS

INTERPRETATION AND INTERVENTION

KAM-SHING YIP

science publishers
New York

Library of Congress Cataloging-in-Publication Data

Names: Yip, Kam-Shing, author.
Title: Drug addiction, trauma and mental illness : interpretation and intervention / Kam-shing Yip (Department of Applied Social Sciences, Hong Kong Polytechnic University, Hong Kong, China).
Description: Hauppauge, N.Y. : Nova Science Publisher's, Inc., [2018] | Series: Psychology research progress | Includes index.
Identifiers: LCCN 2018037645 (print) | LCCN 2018038105 (ebook) | ISBN 9781536140217 (ebook) | ISBN 9781536140200 (hardcover) | ISBN 9781536140217 (ebook)
Subjects: LCSH: Drug abuse. | Drug addiction--Psychological aspects.
Classification: LCC RC564 (ebook) | LCC RC564 .Y57 2018 (print) | DDC 362.29--dc23
LC record available at https://lccn.loc.gov/2018037645

Published by Nova Science Publishers, Inc. † New York

CONTENTS

PREFACE

Substance abuse and drug addiction has long been a problem in our societies. Not to mention numerous people with problems in substance abuse and drug addiction. In addition, there is complexity and comprehensiveness in chronic drug addiction. Many research and clinical experiences tend to point out that people engaging in drug addiction for some years usually embrace severe mental illness, including schizophrenia, borderline personality disorder (BPD), depression, and post-traumatic stress disorder (PTSD). Schizophrenia usually occurs in people with prolonged addiction to amphetamines and hallucinogens. BPD commonly happens in those female addicts with abandonment traumas and abuse in childhood. Depressive mood is co-morbid with the withdrawal effects in chronic drug addiction.

A close look at clients with chronic drug addiction usually reveals that they encounter suffering, hardship, and traumas. There are two types of traumas encountered by people with drug addiction. The first one is trauma before drug addiction and substance abuse. Many of them may have abuse, oppression, and abandonment in life. All these make them feel frustrated, inferior, angry, lonely, and fearful in facing their traumas. Their social support system is thin and inadequate. Substance abuse and drug addiction tends to be the only way to heighten their physical stimulation so that they can escape, suppress, and even repress all this frustration, difficulties, and negative feelings. On the other hand, prolonged drug addiction can also lead to traumas and sufferings, in particular those with chronic drug addiction. The adverse effects of addiction deprive their health, their social functioning, and financial conditions. Many of them become poor and physically and mentally ill.

As a consequence, prolonged drug addiction, severe mental illness, and trauma before and after drug addiction are closely related to one another. Their relationship occurs in several ways. First, drug addiction can serve as a coping mechanism in facing the painful recall and triggering of trauma in life and in addiction. It can also delay the onset of various forms of severe mental illness (Force A). That means, if a person is vulnerable to the onset of schizophrenia because of the breaking effects of trauma and sufferings, drug addiction at least can give them a time to escape or paralyze all these painful breaking effects on the self-system.

Second, the process of chronic drug addiction also provokes related traumas as well as mental problems (Force B). The harmful effects of prolonged drug addiction deteriorates not only the function of the brain and central nervous system but one's physical health. For instance, ketamine has a strong, harmful effect on the bladder. Nearly all drugs pose severe harm to the liver and kidney. Related physical harm actually retards one's social functioning, abilities, and concentration on work, study, recreation, and social interaction, making people with chronic drug addiction become socially, psychologically, and financially deprived and isolated. In addition, in craving for drugs, individuals may even commit illegal and immoral acts, such as sex trade, drug trafficking, drug dealing, and robbery. Finally, in severe drug addiction, one may even have a diffusion of consciousness in which s/he suffers from physical abuse, sex abuse, and bullying by others. All these are painful traumas for people with drug addiction in which various types of mental problems are nurtured. According to related theories of trauma, the breaking effects of traumas on the ego system make the individual becomes vulnerable to the onset of psychosis. The loss of a good object facilitates the individual in having a major depressive disorder. The dissociative effects of trauma certainly speed up the possibility of an anxiety disorder and dissociative disorders.

Within the complexity and intermingling effects of the drug-induced traumas, as well as life traumas, the writer describes interpretation and intervention of clients with trauma, mental illness and chronic drug addiction.

The whole book is divided into four chapters. In chapter 1, the writer outlines challenges faced by related professionals in working with clients with chronic drug addiction. It includes resistance and countertransference of clients toward related workers; intensive emotions and confusion at the rock bottom of chronic addiction; craving for drug and complaints, hopelessness of family members; accumulated traumas, crises, and emergencies in the process of drug addiction as well as related immoral, illegal, and irrational issues together with chronic drug addiction.

In chapter 2, the complexity and comprehensiveness of drug addiction, trauma, and mental illness is mentioned. Different forms of combinations of two Forces A and B are mentioned and elaborated. In addition, how these combinations are related to different types of drugs, traumas, and severe mental illness is fully described. It includes stimulants, anesthetics, hallucinogens, and tranquilizers. For severe mental illness, it includes schizophrenia, depressive disorders, BPD, PTSD, and gender confusion. Regarding traumas, it includes abandonment trauma, physical and sexual abuse, bullying and other forms of oppression. Complexity and comprehensiveness exist in various forms of combinations of trauma, mental illness, and drug addiction. For instance, a female with abandonment trauma usually harbors a feature of BPD and takes stimulants, such as amphetamine. She may regard her boyfriend as a substitute attachment figure to fulfill her attachment hunger. At the same time, the intake of amphetamines may stimulate the recall of her memories of abandonment trauma through drug-induced delusions and hallucinations. Further drug addiction may even induce more traumas and abandonment from the client's substituted attachment figures with a result of intensifying her attachment hunger and abandonment trauma. It certainly becomes a vicious cycle of endless abandonment traumas and drug addiction.

Chapter 3 is a discussion on understanding and intervention for people with drug addiction, abandonment trauma, and BPD. For female clients with chronic drug addiction, many of them suffer from abandonment trauma in their childhood and adolescence. Because of this, they harbor a strong attachment need to substitute attachment figures. However, when they come close to all these substituted attachment figures, their unpleasant memories of being abandoned are triggered. Thus, they have an intimacy crisis in relating to others. On one hand, they have strong attachment hunger to the substituted attachment figures. On the other hand, they harbor fear in intimate relationships. The intimacy crisis makes them fail to establish a suitable degree of intimacy with others. Also, any real or imagined separation from their substituted attachment figures may also arouse their abandonment anger in which they become highly sensitive, irritable, and overreactive to others' slight or mild criticism, ignorance, and non-attention. They easily throw out their anger and frustration. Some may even engage in emotional blackmailing of others by suicidal attempts, self-cutting, reckless driving, and other self-injurious behaviors. Facing all that, related substitute attachment figures may become highly frustrated and finally leave them, making them feel dreadfully lonely and empty. Under that sort of condition, individuals with BPD may easily regard drug addiction as the only substitute attachment figure to gratify their attachment hunger. For many female clients, they may attach to their boyfriends or spouses with chronic drug addiction. To affirm their attachment, they may thus engage in drug addiction together with their spouses or boyfriends. However, prolonged drug addiction also induces related traumas, such as being abandoned by their family members or significant others, as they may crave drugs with severe mental and physical deterioration. That means, on one hand, drug addiction serves as the final substituted attachment object. On the other hand, chronic and severe drug addiction also induces further abandonment trauma that intensifies related symptoms, such as fluctuating emotions, relationships, and self-image in BPD.

In chapter 4, the writer attempts to have a comprehensive interpretation on psychosis and chronic drug addiction. Related literature shows that chronic drug addiction is closely related to the onset of schizophrenia or vice versa. As mentioned above, people with chronic drug addiction are vulnerable to the onset of schizophrenia, in particular those addicted to amphetamine, hallucinogens, and ketamines. Prolonged stimulating effects of these drugs may contribute to the onset of schizophrenia. In taking amphetamines, individuals feel highly excited and agitated. In doing so, both their physical and mental activities are highly stimulated. Together these can be the occurrence of a flight of ideas such as grandiose delusions and hallucinations. Some individuals may delude that they are superman/woman and can fly out their window. Some may even think that they become cleverer than before with lot of ideas to win horse racing and lotteries. Some become very brave and courageous in performing those duties and activities that they would rarely dare to do so in normal times. A timid man who wants to but dare not chase around a beautiful girl may suddenly become very open and aggressive in initiate courtship. Gradually, individuals are not addicted to taking amphetamine but rather addicted to drug-induced grandiose delusions. As their addiction increases, so does the grandiosity of their drug-induced hallucinations and delusions. It becomes more and more similar to grandiose delusions in schizophrenia. After several years of chronic, heavy, and severe addiction to amphetamines, the occurrence of grandiose delusions occurs automatically even without drug taking.

A similar situation happens in taking hallucinogens, in which favorable visual or auditory hallucinations are induced by the effects of hallucinogens. Individuals addicted to hallucinogens often proclaim that all these drug-induced hallucinations are highly stimulating and gratifying their unfulfilled wishes. A student who looks for good grade in a coming tough examination, after taking marijuana (a kind of hallucinogen), may say that s/he deludes that s/he has already gotten and is enjoying the very good grade in this examination. All these drug-induced hallucinations are very attractive and seductive to related individuals, making them more and more absorbed in that and finally become addicted to hallucinogens. As s/he becomes a chronic user, related hallucinations are highly intensified and fragmented.

Finally, all these hallucinations occur spontaneously even without drug taking. At that moment, a hallucinogen-induced psychosis should be formed. Together with drug-induced traumas, the content of hallucinations may change accordingly from unfulfilled wishes to related traumatic memories.

As an opposite, hallucinogens and amphetamines may, at the same time, deter the onset of psychosis. For those clients with intensive traumas in their childhood and adolescence, they may need intensive psychic and mental energy to repress the triggering and rebound of these traumatic experiences and memories. Otherwise, frequent rebound and triggering of trauma may result in intensive self-breaking. As a consequence, they are vulnerable to self-fragmentation and the onset of schizophrenia. To reactivate related internal psychic and mental energy, these clients may be inclined to taking hallucinogens and amphetamines. Under that sort of condition, drug-induced hallucinations may be highly various among individuals. Some may have grandiose hallucinations with contents of unfulfilled wishes (Type 1). Some may have a triggering of previous traumatic memories (Type 2). Some may have a mixture of both (Type 3). In normal cases, individuals may first have Type 1 hallucination and feel happy about that. Their mental and psychic energy is activated by a delusive actualization of their unfulfilled wishes induced by the drug effects. Under that sort of condition, the onset of psychosis may thus be deterred. Later, as the drug addiction grows and persists, mental and psychic energy activated by drugs exhaust the individual's residual ego strengths and energy. Consequently, the individual's residual energy to suppress his/her traumatic memories is exhausted. Thus, drug-induced hallucinations tend to be Type 2, the triggering of previous traumatic memories. The rebound of these traumatic memories gradually intensifies in forms of paranoid delusions and hallucinations. At that moment, it is actually the onset of schizophrenia. If the client is continuously addicted to amphetamines and hallucinogens, the content of hallucinations may finally be a combination of both Type 1 and Type 2 together. Unfulfilled wishes in Type 1 hallucinations may finally intensify to form grandiose hallucinations. In severe cases, individuals may even change their self-identity to a delusive grandiose identity. A combination of Type 1 and Type 2 may finally produce a shift among paranoid and grandiose delusions and hallucinations.

The situation may be different if the individual is addicted to tranquilizers. The effects of tranquilizers make them feel clam, peaceful, and in many ways detached from the painful, abusive, and oppressive reality in family, community, and society. By doing so, it can deter or delay the onset of schizophrenia. However, the tranquilizing effects of the drug also hinder his/her overall ego and social functioning, making the individual become more and more inert, passive, and withdrawn. That means, their repression mechanism of traumatic memories and experiences increase because of the tranquilizing effects of related drugs. As the addiction of the tranquilizer increases, individuals may finally become highly inert, passive, and withdrawn from reality. That means, s/he may be deeply regressive and unable to perform normal roles in family, work, and social interaction. As social isolation and self-isolation increase, the individual may finally suffer from self-breaking and the onset of schizophrenia. However, the onset does not start with active positive symptoms of schizophrenia, such as prevailing paranoid and/or grandiose delusions and hallucinations. Instead, it may manifest in a form of negative symptoms, such as alogia (difficulties in speech and expression), anhedonia (difficulties in social interaction and search for happiness), avolition (difficulties in meaningful actions and behaviors), and blunted affect (difficulties in having normal affective responses). That means, traumatic repression with the numbing of senses and responses finally turns into intensive regression in which alogia can be regarded as extreme repression of speech and expression; anhedonia can be regarded as extreme repression of social interaction and search for happiness; avolition can be regarded as extreme repression of meaningful actions and behaviors; and blunted affect can be regarded as extreme repression of normal affective responses.

Chapter 1

Challenges in Working with People with Chronic Drug Addiction

Introduction

In this chapter, the writer outlines challenges faced by related professionals in working with clients with chronic drug addiction. It includes resistance and countertransference of clients toward related workers; intensive emotions and confusion at the rock bottom of chronic addiction; craving for drug and complaints, hopelessness of family members; accumulated traumas, crises, and emergencies in the process of drug addiction as well as related immoral, illegal, and irrational issues together with chronic drug addiction.

Challenges in Working with Clients with Chronic Drug Addiction

Clients with chronic addiction are well known to be difficult to work with. They are also heavily indulged in drug taking and deeply absorbed in their drug-stimulated inner world and drug-related peers. Many of them may not be accessible for drug detoxification and recovery services. For those who are accessible to related services, they may be highly resistant and unmotivated. They may be involuntary clients being referred by the police or court, as they have legally been charged in the storage, dealing, and/or taking of drugs. They may think that social workers are unable to help them. They regard social workers and clinical professionals as merely legal agents assigned by the legal system to manage and control them. Some of them are at their rock bottom with poor mental and physical health, as well as personal and financial crises that demand immediate help and intervention from professionals. However, when they work through their rock bottom, they become unmotivated clients. Perhaps the following self-narration from an experienced social worker B may illustrate all these clearly.

> M: I have been working with clients with chronic drug addiction in a rehabilitation center for many years. In no way are our clients voluntary and motivated. Many of them come to our center only when they are at the rock bottom of their lives. Their health is deteriorating. Their mental state is unstable. Their financial condition is poor. They have nowhere to go. I remember I had a client A. She was a young adult around twenty-five years old but had been addicted to amphetamines for ten years already. In the past, she was young and beautiful. But after ten years' history in taking "ice," she appeared pale, thin, and weak. She also harbored active delusions and hallucinations. She was financially deprived and poor, as all her money was spent in buying drugs. She had no money, no health, and no peers. She came to our center to ask for food, money, and shelter. I helped her to apply for financial assistance and accommodation in a youth hostel. We needed to wait three months to process all these applications. Within this period of time, she was cooperative and thankful for my help. She was frank in sharing her background, life history, and related experiences in drug addiction. She was also very motivated to join a detoxification and recovery group in our center. Her dosage and frequency in drug taking was greatly reduced. Finally, all these applications were successful. She was able to move into a youth hostel. While everything seemed on the right track, two months later, the warden of the youth hostel rung me and said she had not returned to the hostel for three days. No one knew her whereabouts. Later, one client in my center who knew her well

told me that she cohabited with a new boyfriend who was a drug dealer. They both sold and were addicted with ketamines. At that moment, I was very frustrated. All my efforts in these six months were in vain. She simply disappeared and did not appear again. I soon forgot about this client and was absorbed in my work again. One year later, this client appeared again. She was at another rock bottom in her life. She was deeply depressed, as her boyfriend had just left her. She was also in a financial crisis with nowhere to go. She was also deeply absorbed in drug addiction. Once, she took an overdose of ice and nearly took her life. Fortunately, her friend saved her. She had nowhere to go, and that was why she came to visit me again. In fact, I was really sick of her. In her eyes, I was not a respectable social worker but simply a resourceful person for money, accommodation, and other services. When my resources were given and used up, I became useless. She used my referred resources to cheer herself up so that she could be recovered and with enough health, beauty, and attraction to find another boyfriend. Soon after, she engaged in drug addiction again with her new boyfriend.

Resistance and Countertransference

Many people with chronic drug addiction have encountered numerous abandonment traumas in life. As mentioned above, some abandonment traumas occurred within their early life development. Some abandonment traumas were induced by drug addiction. With all these abandonment experiences, on one hand, they tend to hold up their trust of others. On the other hand, they may have a strong urge to attach to others. This approach and avoidance dilemma have a strong impact on the client–worker relationship. When they are in need of the worker's help, they may seem to be highly attached to the worker and earnestly urge for their help. However, they may become highly sensitive to the worker's comments, advice, and separation. A worker who is on a long vacation temporarily transfers their client to another worker, and this may make the client feel that s/he is being abandoned by his/her worker. Thus, to avoid being hurt or separated, many clients with chronic drug addiction appear reluctant and resistant to a worker's help. However, deep down in their mind, they are, in fact, looking earnestly for acceptance, support, and even caring by the worker. That sort of approach and avoidance complex may exist in a form of countertransference and resistance in the intervention process. It may manifest in the following ways:

1. Being highly critical to a worker's help, ideas, guidance, and advice
2. Turning away and absence of direct eye contact in the interview
3. Loss of contact or sudden withdrawal in the intervention process
4. Missing appointment or frequently late to appointments
5. Outburst of intensive anger toward worker
6. Manifestation of intense negative emotions

In facing all these, social workers need to be highly patient and accepting. If they remain genuine, helpful, and warm, sooner or later, their clients with chronic drug addiction may show appreciation and intensive attachment to them. However, once this intensive attachment is affirmed, the clients may be over attached to the therapist and be highly sensitive to further slight rejection, criticism, and comment.

Intensive Emotions and Confusion

Prolonged and chronic drug addiction is a painful process in which the individual encounters, absorbs, and even represses a great deal of suffering, frustration, and trauma in his/her life. In normal circumstances, it would be quite difficult for him/her to air out such difficulties, traumas, and frustration, as most of their significant others have abandoned or separated from him/her in the process of chronic drug addiction. The presence of a genuine and supportive caregiver or a therapist with comforting and caring words certainly offers an excellent way to air out all these deep-down repressed difficulties and frustrations. That is why once s/he encounters a caring and empathic worker, is it so easy to air out all their frustration and long-suppressed negative emotions and confusion in life. Another reason for the intensive emotion and confusion is that clients with chronic drug addiction, after taking a high dosage of drugs, always become confused in forms of intensive excitement, subconscious out-of-body experiences, or absorbed in drug-induced hallucinations and delusions. In doing so, their long-repressed negative emotions and traumatic memories are easily aroused and rebound. Therapists or anyone close to them would become the first ones to feel their intensive negative emotions and a highly confused mind.

Craving for Drugs

For people with chronic drug addiction, accessibility or obtaining drugs is always their first priority in life. Since they have mentally and physically deteriorated, their social functioning is greatly hindered. Many of them become poor, unemployed, and/or expelled and isolated from their friends, colleagues, and family members. On one hand, they are poor and deprived. On the other hand, they need money earnestly and urgently to buy their drugs for the regular and increasingly intensive addiction. They crave drugs so as to paralyze or escape from deteriorating mental and physical health, as well as the cruel and painful reality and frustration in life. To get the money for regular drug use, many of them may commit illegal offenses and/or immoral deeds, such as drug dealing, sex trade, robbery, shoplifting, or betraying their friends and relatives. Some even borrow money from loan sharks or are heavily indebted. All these make their life, body, and mind become highly confused and messy. With this are the prevailing negative emotions, including worthlessness, helplessness, meaninglessness, and loneliness. Within these conditions, life for them is merely severe addiction and endless pain. That is why many people with chronic drug addiction intend to end their painful and addictive life by various forms of self-harm, suicide, and/or taking an overdose of drugs. It is highly complicated for related professionals to face clients' suicide, illegal offenses, immoral behaviors, and huge debt from loan sharks. They should not just provide psychological counseling, but also legal and financial advice, psychiatric emergencies, and crisis intervention for clients with chronic drug addiction. This is highly emotional laborious work. Related professionals may easily become tense, anxious, and confused in the process of intervention. As a consequence, they easily become fatigued and burnt out after years of highly demanding and intensive work with clients with chronic drug addiction. Below is the self-narration from a social worker who has been working with clients with drug addiction for many years. Related parties' consensus in using their stories for academic purposes was sought. To ensure confidentiality, their personal information and identity was properly disguised.

> Social Worker Q: I have been working with clients with chronic drug addiction in a drug rehabilitation center for around twelve years. Indeed, I feel tired and exhausted both physically and mentally. It is really hard to work with clients with chronic drug addiction. First of all, they are highly fluctuating in their emotions. When they crave drugs, they are emotionally unstable. When they have taken drugs, they seem to be mentally and emotionally stable. Most of them harbor many life frustrations, but it's being covered by drug addiction. One time, they cover them up when they have enough money to take drugs and when their mental and physical conditions are stable. Another time, they beg for your mercy and throw out their hardships and difficulties in life. They urge you for all kinds of assistance, including financial, housing, and medical consultation, as well as psychological comfort and physical togetherness.
>
> In addition to all these, they may suddenly ring up saying that they are going to commit suicide by jumping into the sea or taking a dangerous dosage of drugs because life is too hard and too empty for them. Being a social worker, you have to cater all their needs regardless of time and the situation. It is really too demanding for us. I remember once at home, I was sleeping soundly. My supervisor rang me up saying my client had rung our hotline service saying she was ready to jump into the sea to committing suicide because her boyfriend had just broken up with her. At that moment, she had taken a heavy dosage of hallucinogens. The situation was risky, and she yelled for my immediate companionship and emotional ventilation. I had no choice but immediately got out of bed and rushed to the client's situation.

There were already policemen and many observers there. I had to deliver immediate counseling. Of course, it was highly demanding and stressful to me. If this occurred frequently, of course I would be emotionally, physically, and mentally overloaded.

After years of intensive and emotionally laborious work, I felt mentally and physically exhausted. I suffered from insomnia, psychosomatic symptoms, and irritable bowel symptoms. I easily got sick. I was also so anxious and terrified to receive a phone call from clients. For two years, I was unable to work as a social worker in the center. I needed to change my work to be a social worker in an elderly center. I got tired of encountering young clients, in particular those with emotional problems, behavioral problems, and/or chronic drug addiction.

Within these two years, I was able to have a good rest and began to reflect on what I had done in working with clients with chronic drug addiction. I knew that I did accumulate a lot of wisdom in working with them. I knew how to talk to them and establish a good rapport with them. I knew how they felt in prolonged drug addiction. I knew how to help them to review their life and motivate them to share their suffering with others. However, I was involved with them too much. I needed to remind myself to keep a reasonable distance. Also, their situations severely fluctuated. When they enjoyed their drugs, they forgot about you. When they craved drugs and when they were in their rock bottom, they clung to you. When they had adhered to drugs and drug-related peers, they would depart from us. They would not appear. Knowing all that, I began to be more at ease with their response. When they departed from us, I knew that sooner or later when they had troubles they would return. When they adhered closely to us, I knew that sooner or later when they got what they wanted, they would run away. With all that, I felt more relaxed. I began to accumulate my former experiences in working with clients with chronic drug addiction.

Complaints and Hopelessness of Family Members

For people with chronic drug addiction, their physical and social functioning is not only severely impaired by drug addiction, but their interpersonal relationships, in particular family relationships, are also deeply destroyed. When they crave drugs, they may even steal money from their family, abandon their family, and abuse their family members.

For those supportive family members, initially, they may harbor intensive hope that sooner or later their loved ones may abstain from chronic drug addiction. At first, within the family members' support, clients with drug addiction may voluntarily go to the rehabilitation center for drug detoxifications. However, because of various reasons, many of them relapse frequently within a vicious cycle of drug addiction, detoxification, and relapse again. Gradually, the hope of their family members is shattered. The clients crave drugs, tell lies, and betray their family members. Facing all that, related professionals become the only ones family members can turn to and lodge their complaints and share their frustration. For some highly emotional family members, they may also project their anger toward related professionals affirming that their detoxification, rehabilitation programs, and counseling are not effective. That is why clients' drug addiction turns worse.

Furthermore, for some clients with prolonged chronic drug addiction, they have already lost contact with their family members. To avoid being betrayed by clients with drug addiction, to avoid being labeled as a family of drug addiction, some family members purposefully move away and refuse to have any linkage with clients anymore.

They affirm that clients with chronic drug addiction are hopelessness and can never return back to normal or recover. The situation is even more complicated for those addictive families in which two or more family members engage in various forms of drug addictions. On one hand, family members influence one another in drug addiction. On the other hand, they complain to one another in prolonged drug addictions. In all these cases, drug addiction intermingles with complicated family dynamics and conflicts.

It is highly complicated and difficult for related professionals to tackle all these in the process of intervention.

Accumulated Traumas, Crises, and Emergencies

As mentioned above, prolonged drug addiction involves accumulated traumas, crises, and emergencies. Many of these traumas or crises are, in fact, induced by drug addiction. In the process of drug-related counseling and interventions, related professionals have to face spontaneous challenges from clients' self-harm, such as reckless driving, self-cutting, suicidal ideation and attempts as well as overdosage of drugs. All these mean endless crises and psychiatric emergencies that should be out of the abilities and capacities of related professionals. Some empathic professionals may easily become mentally and physically exhausted in facing all these endless crises and emergencies. They may be professionally burnt out, or some may suffer from various kinds of psychosomatic disorders, such as migraines, irritable bowel symptoms, and anxiety disorders. Some may even feel highly detached and dissociated in facing their clients with endless crises and emergencies. As a consequence, some even feel highly exhausted in working with clients with chronic drug addiction.

Immorality, Illegality, and Irrationality

For people with chronic drug addiction, because of cravings for money for drugs, they may commit various kinds of immoral and illegal activities, such as drug dealing, sex trade, and other criminal activities. Facing all that, they may have to face criminal charges and moral sanctioning from related parties. Some commit illegal and immoral offenses when they are mentally confused by the effects of heavy dosage of drugs. For instance, some males, under the effects of alcohol and amphetamines, may commit sex offenses toward females. Some may engage in gang fights, shoplifting, and robbery. Because of all that, many people with chronic drug addiction may be sentenced to imprisonment or detention in corrective institutions. All these create further complications and complexities for psychosocial intervention for people with chronic drug addiction. On one hand, related professionals have to face the dynamic and complex legal system to intervene for clients with chronic drug addiction. On the other hand, they have to concern related traumas induced to the clients in the legal system and corrective institution. All these create extra burdens and difficulties in psychosocial intervention for clients with chronic drug addiction. The following self-narration from an experienced social worker clearly demonstrates such difficulties and challenges in detail. Related parties' consensus in using their stories for academic purposes was sought. For the sake of confidentiality, their personal identities and information are properly disguised.

> K said the following: I have been an experienced social worker in a drug addiction counseling center for twelve years. I have worked with different types of clients with various kinds of drug addiction. The most difficult part of my job is that I have to face clients' illegal, immoral, and indecent acts in their chronic drug addiction. Once, one of my clients committed a drug-dealing offense. The police approached me to ask for criminal evidence for this offense. It was really a professional dilemma.
>
> On one hand, I was obliged by law to disclose my client's situation to the policeman, as this client was put under the court procedures. On the other hand, as a professional social worker, I needed to keep strict confidentiality for my client. I told my supervisor about my situation. He was not able help much. He simply insisted I keep the confidentiality of my client. Finally, I found my way out. I told my client that the police approached me to obtain criminal evidence and that anything he wanted to tell the police I would repeat it.
>
> On another occasion, one of my clients was caught by the police within the police station; I had to escort her out. The whole night was so dreadful for me. She kept on asking me how to deal with the police. She insisted that I lie and say that at the time of the illegal offense, she was with me at the center. I had to be a witness of her presence in our center. It really disturbed me a lot, as I had to tell a lie. If the police knew that I gave false evidence, I would probably be legally charged and sent to prison. I affirmed that I should not give any false evidence to the police. She threatened me, saying that if I did so, she would be charged with drug dealing and then imprisoned. Instead of imprisonment, she'd rather die immediately by committing suicide in front of me. She tried to run out to the main road and let a truck or bus run her over. I pulled her to stay with me. She struggled hard to free from my control. It was really embarrassing for me; I was a

young adult male, and she was a female youth. People around could have wrongly concluded that I was her boyfriend, and we had were having a fight. Finally, I agreed to give the false evidence to the police. Fortunately, the police did not discover that and, one year later, she committed another illegal drug dealing. She was sentenced to three years imprisonment.

The above-mentioned case clearly shows related difficulties in working with clients with chronic drug addiction with immoral and illegal offenses. Related professionals easily engage in conflicts of giving legal evidence for police with the risk of bridging confidentiality. They may be threatened by clients to give false court evidence of being innocent in legal offenses. Facing all that, some clients may also emotionally and mentally collapse in the court and legal process. That means, related professionals have to accompany them to go through all these processes, which means extra professional input and obligation in the intervention.

PROFESSIONAL ATTRIBUTES IN WORKING WITH CLIENTS WITH CHRONIC DRUG ADDICTION

Facing all the above-mentioned challenges in working with clients with chronic drug addiction, it is crucial that related professionals can possess the following attributes in intervention.

Clinical Supervisor and Colleagues' Support

As clients with chronic drug addiction are highly complicated and dynamic, related professionals should receive good clinical support from their supervisor and colleagues. Clinical support is crucial in particular for those young and inexperienced workers. They are easily frustrated by the crises, emergency, traumas, and resistance from clients with chronic drug addiction. Many of young professionals fail to recognize the specific nature of chronic drug addiction. They need to be trained and equipped with different models and perspectives in interventions with clients with chronic drug addiction. They need support from seniors in dealing with clients' drug-induced traumas and deteriorating mental and physical conditions. For those professionals who also have personal and/or professional traumas in their life, they need to be supported by their colleagues emotionally and clinically. Furthermore, clients with chronic drug addiction are skillful in manipulating related professionals. Below is a self-narration by a social worker in a drug rehabilitation center showing how a female client with chronic drug addiction arouses conflicts and dynamics among workers and clients. Related parties' consensus to use their stories for academic purposes were sought, and for the sake of confidentiality, their personal information and identity were properly disguised.

> Q: I had been a social worker in a drug rehabilitation center for more than twelve years. This was a residential care center for female adolescents and adults with drug addiction. They lived in our center for six months for rehabilitation. Apart from proper detoxification from drugs, they needed to learn some occupational skills, such as word processing, shorthand, or hair design so that they could earn a living after discharge. It was highly dynamic in looking down all these adolescents with drug addiction. Many of them harbored many traumas in life, such as being abandoned, abused, or oppressed by their caregivers. Some were involved in the sex trade, drug trafficking, and dealing. Many of them were emotionally unstable and impulsive. Some had several abortions within five years. They were highly dynamic, irritable, and easily provoked by trivial interpersonal matters. Mary was a young person who had a drug addiction for five years and was involved in the sex trade and drug dealing for two years. She was sentenced by the court to come to this center for detoxification and rehabilitation.
>
> When Mary first entered the center, she was highly resistant and defensive. She thought that our colleagues had cooperated with her probation office to watch over her. She did not say much. She was highly aggressive and manipulative. When other residents said any negative words against her, she would throw a tantrum and curse them. Sometimes, it might end up with a fight. When our colleagues, in particular me who was her responsible social worker, approached her for counseling, she kept quiet and did not look at us. She was impolite, unmotivated, and highly

rebellious in residential life. Her probation officer warned her if she failed to be cooperative in residential life, she would be sent back to prison for her drug dealing and sex trade.

At that moment, she began to adapt to residential life but still thought that other female residents were simple and childish in comparison to her rich life experiences. She also thought that she was the most attractive and beautiful woman in the residential center. She even tried to seduce other residents' boyfriends and brothers. All this made other residents become highly aggressive. They grouped together and pushed Mary to leave the center. However, at the same time, Mary fully knew that our center was in charge and that Joey was the final authority at the center. She came to her office in tears and begged for her mercy. She fully appreciated Joey's professionalism and caring attitude. She bowed down for her mercy and stayed at the center. From that time onward, Joey became Mary's shelter from residents' attacks. Mary was also very clever in stirring up anger among residents. She provoked their anger among one another. She told Resident A her how another Resident B hated her and vice versa. The same tactics were used to arouse conflicts and dynamics among colleagues. Her tactics were highly successful in removing those residents and colleagues she disliked. One year later, three colleagues resigned and around six residents left the houses.

The center in charge finally acknowledged that she could not keep and protect Mary anymore. At the same time, Mary's duration in staying in this center had been fulfilled. She needed to be discharged. At this stage, Mary thought that we were going to abandon her. Facing all that, she was going to be impulsive and manipulative to manifest her abandonment, fear, and anger. Together with this were the frequent self-harming tactics from self-cutting to suicidal gestures. She purposefully threw out her anger by intending to jump off from the window ledge. One night, she swallowed a huge dosage of sleeping pills and cut her wrist so as to die immediately. We had no choice but send her to a nearby hospital for immediate psychiatric treatment. From that time onward, we dared not to admit her back to the rehabilitation center. Instead, she was sent to a mental hospital with a complicated diagnosis of borderline personality disorder, suicide, and self-harm.

Advanced Professional Training

Clients with chronic drug addiction are difficult clients with highly complicated traumas. They are also highly resistant with emotional blackmailing behaviors as well as suicide and self-harm. Many of them even harbor various forms of severe mental illness, such as schizophrenia, major depressive disorder, and BPD. All these imply that related professionals need to have advanced professional training in dealing with clients with chronic drug addiction. Advanced professional training implies knowledge and skills in working with severe mental problems including schizophrenia, suicide, major depressive disorder and BPD. It also includes various perspectives and knowledge of counseling persons with different types of traumas. Only with all this equipment can related professionals develop their professional competence in working with clients with chronic drug addiction. Furthermore, comprehensive and advanced professional training enables workers to develop their practice wisdom in a well-guided way without committing too much failure that diminishes their professional image and competence. Finally, advanced professional training induced by senior scholars or specialist also implies ongoing well-structured clinical supervision for professionals in working with clients with chronic drug addiction.

Professional Commitment and Endurance

As mentioned above, clients with chronic drug addiction are resistant, complicated, and difficult to deal with. Related professionals need to be persistent, enduring, and committed. Without persistence and endurance, related professionals are easily frustrated by clients' resistance and critical comments. Without commitment to the welfare of clients, related professionals easily become apathetic in facing clients' continuous endless demands at their rock bottom of chronic drug addiction. For many young and green professionals, even though they have good commitment to clients' welfare, they are easily frustrated by clients' resistance and critical comments. They may even feel confused about clients' complexity of traumas and mental illnesses in chronic drug addiction. Some inexperienced workers may even be betrayed by "professional" clients, saying that they are really motivated to abstain from drugs, when in fact they are not.

Humanity, Versatility, Complexity, and Flexibility

Many clients with chronic drug addiction are sophisticated and complicated. They have encountered various traumas in life. They have encountered many people, in particular those with drug addiction and those who deal drugs. Some even participate in illegal and immoral drug dealing and sex trade. Being equipped with all these life experiences, clients with chronic drug addiction may be cunning, highly testing, sophisticated, ambivalent, and complicated. They are professional clients; they know how to manipulate and control workers, as their life experiences are far more complicated and sophisticated than related professionals. For those workers with comprehensive life experiences, in particular those coming from a lower-class background, they may be versatile and complex enough to understand the comprehensiveness of clients with chronic drug addiction. However, for those workers with thin life experiences, especially those who are young and come from a middle-class background, without any rich experiences in encountering people in low-class natures, they may be easily misled or even threatened by clients with chronic drug addiction. It is important that they can develop their humanity, versatility, complexity, and flexibility so that they can have effective intervention with clients with chronic drug addiction.

Humanity means that related professionals should firmly believe that underlying the complexity, cunningness, and resistance of clients with BPDs there are numerous tortures, sufferings, traumas, and unfulfilled needs in their life.

All these need to be understood and cared about by related professionals. It can be developed by getting a detailed life history from clients in the process of intervention. If the clients refuse to disclose everything, related professionals should be patient and wait until one day when clients are ready to do so, in particular at times of their rock bottoms.

Versatility implies that related professionals should be highly versatile in understanding and interacting with clients with chronic drug addiction. The traditional way of interviewing clients within an interview room in fact may not be appropriate in working with clients with chronic drug addiction. At their rock bottom, they need a decent job in which the employer can accept their drug addiction background.

They need to build up their normal social circle through normal social and recreational activities. For some young adult clients, they need to be involved in various types activities that interest them, so as to regain their sense of meaning in life and self-confidence in the process of rehabilitation and recovery. In doing so, related professionals need to be highly versatile with different types of exposure and recreation as well as social interest. It is not surprising to note that a worker who is a good street dancer can attract a group of adolescents with drug addiction for recovery. Once clients join in street dancing training with good social recognition by participating in certain public shows or winning certain competitions, their self-confidence and meaning in life can be restored. In addition, the dancing group is also a support and healthy social circle. All these are vital for a healthy recovery from chronic drug addiction.

Complexity means that related professionals need to be complicated enough to understand the dialectic and dynamic aspect of the human mind and various kinds of subcultures in our society. Many clients with chronic drug addiction are closely linked to delinquent subcultures, popular entertainment cultures, and illegal underground subcultures. Furthermore, clients with chronic drug addiction are trapped within unresolved emotional complexes, such as inferiority and superiority, love and hate, approach and avoidance complexes toward themselves, others, and drug addiction.

Complexity also applies to clients with different degrees of drug addiction. The natures and characteristics of occasional users, regular users, and chronic users are vastly different. Facing all these complexities, it is highly irrelevant for related professionals to regard professional interventions simply just like a straight forward application of intervention procedures from a protocol-like intervention guideline. Some inexperienced professionals may simply regard drug detoxification or the introduction of destructive effects of various types of drugs as the only models in psychosocial intervention.

In fact, all these highly reductionistic and simplified models are only suitable to occasional drug users in which their habits of drug use are influenced mostly by external factors, such as peer influence and insufficient knowledge about the adverse effects of drugs. For those chronic drug users, their habits of drug use are mostly influenced by internal factors such as senses of satisfaction and frustration in life as well as former traumatic experiences, in particular attachment traumas.

Flexibility implies related professionals should be highly flexible in working with clients with chronic drug addiction. It goes together with complexity and versatility. Related professionals should be accustomed to having interventions within different natural settings and environments, such as the home, club, street, park, and bar, places where people with chronic drug addiction gather. Flexibility also implies patience and endurance to wait for the suitable chance, time, and place to speak the appropriate words for the client with chronic drug addiction.

Putting humanity, complexity, versatility, and flexibility together means that related professionals are able to enrich their knowledge and competence in knowing, interpreting, and intervening with clients with chronic drug addiction within different perspectives, including the meaning of life, self-system, body, and mind, as well as social roles and functioning. In doing so, individuals with substance abuse are not only drug addicts but holistic persons with different dimensions of life. Every client is unique and individualistic. Apart from taking drugs, they are also people with normal urges for a meaningful life, self-respect, dignity, integrity, and responsible contributions to their own families, society, and country. With that sort of articulation, related interventions are no longer deficit-oriented detoxifications nor pointing out how serious their drug addiction is, but bring hope, normality, and integration in their recovery of chronic drug addiction.

Conclusion

The introductory chapter aims at discussing the complexity and challenges of professionals in working with clients with chronic drug addiction. Certainly, clients with chronic drug addiction are complicated, highly resistant, and embrace strong countertransference toward related professionals. They may also harbor strong negative emotions as well as mental confusion in drug taking. They crave drugs and reach their rock bottoms in chronic drug addiction. Their family members feel hopeless and may harbor strong complaints toward related professionals. Facing all that, professional workers needs to be clinically supported by their seniors and colleagues. They also need to be versatile, complex, and highly flexible in using various means in interventions with their clients within different social and physical contexts. They should be committed and with good endurance and persistence in dealing with clients' resistances, low motivations, and fluctuating emotions and mental confusion in chronic drug addiction. Related agencies should provide substantial and advanced professional training so that workers can develop their practice competence in facing clients' mental, physical, emotional, and interpersonal problems in chronic drug addiction, in particular with numerous life traumas.

Chapter 2

DRUG ADDICTION, TRAUMA, AND MENTAL ILLNESS: COMPLEXITY AND COMPREHENSIVENESS

INTRODUCTION

As mentioned above, traumas, mental illness, and drug addiction correlate with one another in the process of chronic drug addiction. In this chapter, the writer tries to outline an initial framework in understanding various combinations of two forces. Force A is the coping of mental problems and stress by means of drug addiction. Force B is how the deteriorating effects of drug addiction may finally induce various forms of traumas and mental illness. In addition to this, how these combinations are related to different types of drugs, traumas, and severe mental illness are fully described. It includes stimulants, anesthetics, hallucinogens, and tranquilizers. For severe mental illness, it includes schizophrenia, depressive disorders, BPD, PTSD, and gender confusion. Regarding traumas, it includes abandonment trauma, physical and sexual abuse, bullying, and other forms of oppression. Complexity and comprehensiveness exist in various forms of combinations of traumas, mental illness, and drug addiction. For instance, a female person with abandonment trauma usually harbors a feature of BPD and takes stimulants such as amphetamine. She may regard her boyfriend as a substitute attachment figure to fulfill her attachment hunger. At the same time, the intake of amphetamines may stimulate the recall of her memories of abandonment trauma through drug-induced delusions and hallucinations. Furthermore, drug addiction may even induce more traumas and abandonment from the client's substituted attachment figures with a result of intensifying her attachment hunger and abandonment trauma. It certainly becomes a vicious cycle of endless abandonment traumas and drug addiction.

DYNAMICS AND DILEMMAS BETWEEN TRAUMAS AND DRUG ADDICTION

Forces A and B

Their relationship can occur in several ways. First, drug addiction can serve as a coping mechanism in facing the painful recall and triggering of trauma in life and in addiction. It can also delay the onset of various forms of severe mental illness (Force A). That means, if a person is vulnerable to the onset of schizophrenia because of breaking effects of trauma and sufferings, drug addiction at least can give them a time to escape or paralyze all these painful breaking effects on the self-system.

Second, the process of chronic drug addiction also provokes related traumas and mental problems (Force B). The harmful effects of prolonged drug addiction deteriorate not only the function of the brain and central nervous system on one hand but one's physical health. For instance, ketamine has a strong harmful effect on the bladder. Nearly all drugs pose severe harm to the liver and kidneys. Related physical harm actually retards one's social functioning, abilities, and concentration on work, study, recreations, and social interaction, making people with chronic drug addiction become socially, psychologically, and financially deprived and isolated. In addition to that, in craving drugs, individuals may even commit illegal and immoral acts, such as a sex trade, drug trafficking, drug dealing, and robbery. Finally, in severe drug addiction, one may even have a diffusion of consciousness in which s/he suffers from physical abuse, sexual abuse, and bullying by others. All these are painful traumas for people with drug addiction, in which various types of mental problems are nurtured. According to related theories of trauma, the breaking effects of traumas on the ego make the individual become vulnerable to the onset of psychosis. The loss of a good object facilitates the individual to have a major depressive disorder. The dissociative effects of trauma certainly speed up the possibility of anxiety disorders and dissociative disorders.

As mentioned above, there are interacting forces between trauma and drug addiction. Force A implies drug addiction is used to cope with pain and the destructive effects of trauma.

Force B is that prolonged drug addiction induces further traumas. These two forces interact and intermingle with one another.

That means, on one hand, drug addiction and substance abuse provide temporary coping and escape for individuals in facing traumas, sufferings, and hardships in life and delay the onset of possible mental problems (Force A). On the other hand, prolonged drug addiction provokes and induces related traumas and imposes physical and mental harm that nurtures the occurrence of severe mental illness (Force B). There are four ways in which these two forces interact with one another. They can be listed as follows:

1. Force A inhibits Force B
2. Force B inhibits Force A
3. Force A reinforces Force B
4. Force A combines with Force B

In the first combination, *Force A inhibits Force B*. It usually occurs when the individual is not too involved in drug addiction. In other words, Force A is active in which drug addiction successfully facilitates the individual to escape and avoid frustration and recall of traumatic memories and experiences. Similarly, the individual is quite cautious and disciplined in drug addiction. S/he may be a regular user. But s/he is fully alert regarding the destructive effects of the drug. So s/he never has an overdosage of drugs. S/he only uses this whenever s/he feels frustrated, depressed, or stressed, and then s/he takes drugs to alleviate his/her negative emotions and triggering of his/her traumatic memories.

In the second combination, *Force B inhibits Force A.* It usually occurs when the individual is at the lowest ebb of his/her chronic and prolonged drug addiction. S/he is actually caught up with all sorts of drug-induced trauma, such as severe poverty, losing one's employment, and being raped and bullied by others, as well as serious harm physically and mentally because of severe drug addiction. At that moment, the individual fully knows that the disastrous effects of drug addiction actually outweighs its coping and escaping effects. S/he actually is aware that continuous drug addiction may finally spoil his/her whole life, including self-esteem, dignity, mental health, physical health, and even his/her own life. Within this final critical awareness, the individual may be aware that s/he needs detoxification or rehabilitation of his/her drug addiction. If professionals and good friends or relatives are available to persuade, encourage, and support the individual, s/he may initiate his/her own process of recovery. However, if there is no support system, the individual may engage in a love and hate, as well as approach and avoid the dilemma. On one hand, the individual really hates his/her own addiction to drugs. On the other hand, drugs seem to be the only means for him/her to temporarily escape and paralyze himself/herself from all these painful conflicts. In some cases, individuals may cry in times of drug addiction. In some cases, the individual may commit suicide by taking an overdose of drugs.

In the third combination, *Force A reinforces Force B.* That means the force of using drugs to adapt to the frustration of life is reinforcing the force of drug-induced traumas or vice versa. That means, the individual has no way out. The drug-induced traumas have not reached the rock bottom. They are still tolerable. The individual is able to take drugs to escape from the frustrating effects caused by the drug addiction. For instance, an individual has recently acknowledged that his bladder function was deteriorated because of the adverse effects of ketamine addiction. He felt extremely upset and nervous. Rather than stop taking ketamines, as he still had a lot of frustration in life that needed to be paralyzed by ketamines, he took a heavy dosage of ketamine so as to cope with the additional frustration of losing function of his bladder and kidneys. This is a nearly desperate position. The individual fully knows that one day drug addiction can finally ruin his/her life, but the current is still tolerable. Thus, drug addiction is the way s/he chooses. Force A reinforces Force B so that the individual still thinks, clings to, and insists that drug addiction is the only way, only addiction and the only alternative in life. S/he is waiting for the forthcoming day of their rock bottom. But it seems that it is too far away in the current moment.

In the fourth combination, *Force A combines with Force B*. It means that the force of using drugs is as a way to escape from life's frustration combines with the force of drug-induced traumas and sufferings. As these forces may inhibit or reinforce one another, the individual is in a state of high confusion. It usually occurs when the individual has taken related drugs, and the effects of the drugs are going to finish. On one hand, the individual is still enjoying the drug-induced, highly stimulated bodily senses so that s/he can have a sense of elation, out-of-body experience, and/or being tranquilized from the painful and oppressive reality. On the other hand, s/he is subconsciously aware that these heightened bodily senses are nearly at their end. What follows would be a more boring, traumatic, and painful reality s/he is going to face. Both feelings are there. The individual is at a stage of ambivalence and confusion. It is also a state of dissociation in which the individual is detached from the painful reality as well as his/her own state of mind, past traumatic memories, and the future emptiness and meaninglessness. Within all these, the individual is fully engaged in his drug-induced subconscious state of ambivalence and uneasiness. For people with full drug addiction, it seems to be the only way for them to temporarily escape from the traumatic past, painful reality, and hopeless future.

Forces A and B in Different Stages of Drug Addiction

All these four combinations occur within the process of drug addiction in the following stages:

Stage 1: Force A Only (Initial or Occasional Users)

It is too early for Force B to occur (when the individual attempts drug addiction and uses it occasionally).

Stage 2: Force A Inhibits Force B (Regular Users: Initial Addiction)

Force B begins to occur as the individual has taken drugs for quite a period of time. However, the adverse and harmful effects are still mild and within an accepting level. The individual uses drugs regularly to cope with his/her life stress, frustration, and trauma.

Stage 3: Force A Combines with Force B (Long-Term Regular Users: Full Addiction)

Force B begins to prevail, resulting in significant physical and mental damage for the individual. Related damages are still tolerable and acceptable for the individual. S/he fully enjoys the drug addiction. S/he is fully involved in the smoothly and paralyzing effects of drugs. Thus, s/he enjoys the effect of drug taking on one hand and is aware of the serious damage in the future on the other hand. S/he feels a bit confused and ambivalent, in particular within the addictive process.

Stage 4: Force A Reinforces Force B (Chronic Addiction)

In Stage 4, Force A reinforces Force B. Related physical and mental damage to clients with drug addiction is very significant and substantial to a degree that their normal ego and social functioning are hindered. It can be problems in employment, education, normal daily interaction, and daily living pattern. Related clients are fully aware that continuous drug addiction could result in severe damage physically, mentally, psychologically, and socially. However, they believe they do not have any way out. They can only cope with that sort of fear and worry by even more intensive and frequent drug addiction. They are simply waiting for the forthcoming of day of hitting rock bottom. But it seems that it is too far away in the current moment.

Stage 5: Force B Inhibits Force A (Rock Bottom of Chronic Addiction)

Force B inhibits Force A implies the rock bottom of chronic drug addiction. As mentioned above, related clients are in the lowest ebb of his/her life with severe poverty, unemployment, being abused, oppressed, and victimized. They have nowhere to go. Their health is deteriorating, and many of them are facing the final day of total failure of their kidneys, bladder, liver, or other severe physical disease. Deep down in their mind, they are fully aware that only immediate detoxification can save them from the accumulated harmful effects of drug addiction. But they do not have enough courage, determination, resources, or support to do so. All they can do is give in to the continuous craving for drugs until the final day comes.

Within these five stages and two interactive Forces A and B, the writer attempts to describe the highly comprehensive and complicated relationship among drug addiction, trauma, and mental illness. Its implication to psychosocial intervention with people with chronic drug addiction is also mentioned.

MULTI-DIMENSIONAL PERSPECTIVE OF DRUG ADDICTION

Disease and Biochemical Models

E. M. Jellinek (1952, 1960) was the first scholar who suggested the disease model to describe drug addiction. Before 1960, the World Health Organization had already regarded alcoholism was a medical problem. Similarly, the American Medical Association asserted that alcoholism was a treatable illness in 1956. Following this, in 1965, the American Psychiatric Association used the term “disease” to describe alcoholism.

> The aggressive, feeling of guilt, remorse, resentments, withdrawal, etc., which develop in the phases of alcohol addiction, are largely consequences of the excessive drinking…these reactions to excessive

> drinking—which have quite a neurotic appearance—give the impression of a "alcoholic personality."… (Jellinek 1952: 682)

This model assumes people with drug addiction as weak and inadequate that need to be hospitalized, detoxified, and medicated in mental hospitals or detoxification center.

The biochemical model described the harmful effects of various types of drugs on human bodies. According to their pharmacological effects on human bodies, addictive drugs can be divided into the following types:

1. Pain killers
2. Stimulants
3. Tranquilizers
4. Marijuana
5. Hallucinogens

Liska (1990) briefly describes the biochemical effects of these five types of drug as follows:

> For *pain killers*, the most common ones are morphine and heroin. Narcosis is defined as the depression of the central nervous system (brain and spinal cord) leading to analgesia, drowsiness, changes in mood, mental clouding, apathy, lethargy and ultimately unconsciousness.… Morphine has the ability to relieve severe pain without causing loss of consciousness…Heroin…is an excellent pain reliever, long considered by some to more effective than morphine.… (Liska 1994: 147)

> For *cocaine*, it blocks reuptake of NE from synaptic junctions and stimulators release of dopamine. For *amphetamines*, it blocks catecholamine, reuptake, promotes release of dopamine, and directly stimulates receptors. (Liska 1994: 127)

> Cocaine has two main pharmacological actions. It is a powerful CNS stimulant, and an effective local anesthetic with its own vasoconstrictive action.…Modern users describe cocaine's central effects as the "perfect

illusion." They think they are more competent, smarter, sexier, vigilant, masterful, confident, productive and full of energy. (Liska 1994: 174)

In low to moderate oral doses (1–50 mg) *amphetamines* generally have the following effects:

1. Sensation of the CNS
2. Delay the onset of fatigue and the need for sleep
3. Increase blood pressure
4. Increase respiration rate
5. Raise blood or sugar level
6. Dilate the bronchi
7. Divert blood flow from internal organs to skeletal muscle
8. Constrict nasal mucous membranes
9. Depress the appetite
10. Improve athletic performance. (Liska 1994: 185)

When we refer to *minor tranquillizers*, we mean primarily the benzodiazepines....I constitute the main group of drugs for the control of anxiety neuroses. They are also prescribed for tension, muscle spasm, skin rashes, alcohol withdrawal, alcoholism, agitation, hallucinations and convulsions and frequency for insomnia. Benzodiazepine receptors are located predominantly—if not exclusively—in the brain, which explains why benzodiazepines have no action on other tissues such as heart and skeletal muscle. The brain receptors are in the limbic region (the part that deals with emotional regulation and control) and are quite specific; no other drugs bind to these receptors. Benzodiazepines probably act as anti-anxiety, anti-insomnia and anti-convulsant agent by virtue of their ability to facilitate GABA function. (Liska 1994: 256)

The word, hallucinogen, described drug in small doses could alter perception, thought, and mood, creating illusions in the mind of the user. (Liska 1994: 289)

The common types are LSD, PCP, Methaqualone, and Hallucinogenic Amphetamine Derivative (Liska 1994).

Together with this model is also knowledge of long-term harmful effects on various kinds of drugs on human bodies, in particular on one's mental and physical conditions, such as prolonged damage on the central nervous system, lungs, kidneys, and bladder. Being equipped with all this biochemical knowledge, related professionals presumed that long-term harmful effects of various kinds of drugs can serve as a way to educate clients to abstain from long-term and chronic drug addiction. Nevertheless, most regular and chronic users are fully aware of these harmful effects on their bodies and minds. They still adhere to drug addiction because of unresolved emotional complexes and traumas in life.

Harm Reduction Model

The harm reduction approach aims to eradicate or minimize the immediate and long-term harmful effects of drugs on human bodies. Blume and Logan (2013) have summarized several harm reduction approaches as the following:

> Harm reduction approaches are strategies that are used to reduce the harmful consequences of addictive behaviors. Harm reduction often includes multiple approaches including pharmacological, psychological and environmental interventions, designed to reduce risky behaviors and their consequences. (Blume and Logan 2013: 633)

Harm Reduction by Prescribed Controlled Substance

Prescribed controlled substances, usually benzodiazepines, have been used to reduce the discomfort of withdrawal symptoms. The harm reduction pharmacological approach can be described as follows:

> Recent pharmacological advanced have been used successfully to reduce potential harm from substance abuse. Opiate agents such as naltrexone, as well other types of substances (such as acamprosate), have been used to successfully reduce substance-related cravings in many patients.

> Certain depressant drugs…have been used similarly to control mood-triggered substance used with anxiety and depression. In addiction. Recently vaccinations have been used with some success to interfere with psychoactive properties (inhibiting the high) of certain substance of abuse to dissuade further use. (Blume and Logan 2013: 634–5)

It is a strategy that uses “less evil to replace the evil.” Individual clients are encouraged to use another substituted less harmful substance/drug to replace the harmful addicted drug. The physical dependence of the addicted drug is eased out, but the psychological urge to take drugs is still there.

Behavioral Harm Reduction Strategies

Behavioral harm reduction strategies assume that the individual has a strong internal self-control mechanism to control his/her drug addiction. Once, his/her insight of the harmful effects of drug addiction is restored, with others’ help, this internal self-control mechanism can be developed. Behavioral methods such as check and count to times of addiction, alternating addictive behaviors to other behaviors, and switching from high-risk to low-risk addiction are suggested (Blume and Logan 2013). In clinical practice, most regular and chronic users of drugs fully recognize the harmful effects of drug addiction, but it is their only way to escape from the painful reality and frustration in life. Unless their life frustration can be enlightened, behavioral harm reduction is ineffective for them.

Cognitive Harm Reduction Strategies

Cognitive strategy in harm reduction is to challenge the client’s positive expectation and cognition of substance abuse.

> Positive expectancies are the beliefs that clients have about the positive effects or outcomes related to the addictive behavior. Common positive expectancies involve beliefs that the addictive behavior will contribute to increased socialization, power, sexuality, and euphoria. (Blume and Logan 2013)

The therapist challenges clients' irrational beliefs of positive experiences in drug addiction. It presumes that clients with substance abuse have self-control to regulate their own cognitive expectation of substance abuse. However, in clients with drug addiction, especially those with chronic addiction, they are not addicted to the drug but drug-induced subjective experiences, such as euphoria, out-of-body experiences, excitement, and tranquilizing peacefulness helping them to be away from painful feelings and oppressive reality. That means, cognitive harm reduction strategies can help clients with a supportive social environment and with a good self-control mechanism.

Lifestyle Balance Activities

Lifestyle balance activity is also a harm reduction approach in the recent decade. Related workers or life coaches examine clients' lifestyle to check whether they spend appropriate time in different domains in life such as family life, physical self-care, emotional self-care, spirituality, recreation, and social life. It assumes that distress comes from spending too much time in one domain and neglecting the others. Clients are facilitated to have good nutrition, sleep, and exercise as well as medical care. It assumes that as healthy life habits are restored with an improvement in health and mental conditions, clients' dependence on drug addiction can be alleviated. Similar to other harm reduction strategies, this one is effective for clients with a good self-control mechanism, strong resolve, and a good sense of reality, which enable them to change their living habits and reduce their drug addiction accordingly. This approach may be suitable for clients with mild drug addiction, such as using sleeping bills or minor tranquilizers. For them, a balanced lifestyle with more time in recreation, social activities, and good food certainly lowers their anxiety levels and improves their sleeping habits with a reduction in the use of sleeping pills. However, for those heavy and regular users of severe psychoactive substances, such as ketamines, amphetamines, and heroin, they harbor many life frustrations and traumas that need to be repressed by drugs, so this approach is too superficial and ineffective for them.

Existential Perspective

The above-mentioned perspective fails to address the complexity of human life. They presume that the complexity of the human mind and body in drug addiction can be articulated in reductionistic and simplified measurement and controlled by a physical and mental mechanism. They ignore that human beings continuously strive for meaning and sense of existence in life. Most clients with chronic drug addiction feel empty and meaningless in their life endeavors. All these imply that it is crucial to have an existential perspective in understanding and perceiving addiction.

Existential Perspective in Terms of Choice and Meaning

Within existentialism, clients with drug addictions are not passively addicted to drugs. They are people with value and responsibility and harbor a strong will to meaning (Frankl 1997). It is a kind of deep meaning of suffering and love. Clients with drug addiction and substance abuse are deprived of a meaning in life, love, and sufferings. Drug addiction becomes their immediate and preferable choice to repress the senses of meaninglessness and existential frustration.

Psychodynamic Perspective in Drug Addiction

There are many prominent scholars in the psychodynamic perspective, such as Freud, Klein, Bowlby, Winnicott, Sullivan, and Kohut. However, their prime interest is not on drug addiction. Related scholars tried to apply related theories from these prominent figures in understanding the intervention of drug addiction.

Self-Psychology in Drug Addiction: Narcissism and Narcosis

According to Kohut's self-psychology, Ulman and Paul (2006) suggest a Narcissus' model in drug addiction. It has four components:

1) A phenomenology of addiction of what is addiction

> 2) An etiology and pathogenesis of addiction or when are the origins and where are the developmental pathways leading to addiction
> 3) A typology of addiction or who are the various types of addiction
> 4) A therapeutics of addiction or how does a psychotherapist work psychotherapeutically with an addiction pattern. (Ulman and Paul, 2006: xiv)

Ulman and Paul (2006) describe narcissism and narcosis as follows:

> Narcissism and narcosis may be compared like this: in case of narcissism an archaic form of self-love function like a narcotic drug that induces a state of enraptured self-absorption: whereas in the case of narcosis, a drug or other substance produces a narcissistic state of bliss characterized by an ecstatic trance and euphoric obliviousness. (Ulman and Paul, 2006: 4)

Ulman and Paul (2006) affirmed that narcotic drug addiction is a kind of self-love in which the individual is absorbed in a state of an ecstatic trance and euphoric obliviousness. In other words, people with drug addiction are not addicted to the drug. Rather, they are addicted to drug-induced experiences. This is the addictive experience that gratifies the individual's need of egocentric focus and self-love. This sort of self-love theoretically originated from Kohut's self-object relationship. Addictive objects, in many ways, can be regarded as transitional objects for the individual to compensate insufficient caregivers' concerns in early development.

> Ulman and Paul (2006) employ an empathetic introspective stance from Kohut as a means to gaining access to the unconscious fantasy lives of our addicted patients. We discover that unconsciously they are organized in terms of a specific type of archaic does not reinvest the narcissistic capital, which is originally derived from early caregivers, back into nonhuman being things or activities (that is a transitional object) as well as later human caregivers. (Ulman and Paul 2006: xiv)

Khantzian's Self-Medication

Khantzian (1980, 1981) affirmed that drug addiction is actually a matter of self-choice. Everyone chooses his/her own type of drug according to his/her own unfulfilled needs and personality.

> Most substance dependent individual prefers and self select a particular drug. This preference and selection is the result of the drug of choice and its distinctive psychopharmacologic effects interacting with the unique personality organization and reactive patterns of an individual that predisposes a person to dependency on a particular drug. (Khantzian 1980: 32)

For people in narcotic addiction, he concluded that they need the opiates to give them a sense of a dysphoric ego state so that they can overcome sense internalized anger and rage. It also gives them ways to escape from his/her elated depression.

Compulsiveness of Drug Addiction

People with drug addiction embrace a psychological compulsion toward drugs. Glasscote and others (1971) stressed the following:

> By contrast to the term psychological dependence, compulsion is a more specific term that connotes one of the greatest obstacles successfully treating people who have abused drugs. Compulsivity can be manifested in practically any aspect of behavior....
>
> Compulsivity is believed to commonly underlie any number of widespread behavior problems, such as overeating, heavy use of alcohol, gambling, and so on. It seems certain that some portion of those who use illegal drugs do so out of compulsion. This significance is this: compulsions are notably resistant to presently known methods of treatment; the long-term success rate is low, the relapse rate is high. (Glasscote et al. 1972: 55)

In the life history and the direct experience of every patient dependent upon physically addicting drugs, we may discern three layers of compulsion:

a) Acute Withdrawal

The compulsiveness of physical dependency based on entirely on processes on the level of the cells. (The compulsive need to continue with drug to avoid the very uncomfortable feeling of acute withdrawal. This is a strictly physical problems)

b) Protracted Withdrawal

The compulsiveness of protracted withdrawal, a gray area in theory (Addicts who have been withdrawn and are not physically dependent anymore, typically show a persistent longing to return to the drug. This urge or desire is known to endure years, even decades, of enforced abstinence.)

c) Emotional Need

The emotional compulsiveness leading first to start drug use and then to continue the search of effect. Only this third form will be encountered in compulsive users of drugs which are not also physically addictive, like psychedelics or stimulants.

Every neurotic compulsion is viewed as outcomes of a conflict of several incompatible wishes and fears, a conflict which is forcibly pushed out, and kept out, of consciousness. It is characteristic of such compulsions that the more they are lived out in outer reality, the more insatiable they become; it is as if they were continually searching for their real, though unconscious, aim without ever being able to attain it—precisely because the real aim of the wish is buried.

Under any psychological or physiological stress, the compulsion to take drugs (or to show other forms of symptoms) increases. In turn it can be observed that the emotional dependency on the drug is overcome if the psychological dependency and commitment is displaced onto other objects, e.g., to a concrete community, to a cause, or to a therapist. In other words, potent meaning giving factors can replace in highly motivated individuals the compelling role the drug exerts.

Wurmser (1978) described that people are compulsive to drug addiction. There are three types of compulsiveness. The first one is actual physical compulsiveness with acute withdrawal. Clients take drugs to ease up their withdrawal symptoms. The second one is protracted withdrawal with a delayed sense of compulsiveness. The client embraces a lengthened sense of physical withdrawal.

S/he is highly eager to return to the drug. The third one is emotional need. It is a mixture of fear, desires, and intense frustration. As an opposite to Khantzian's self-medication, in Wurmser's (1978) compulsiveness, clients do not have choice. Instead they are compulsive objects controlled by drug addiction. The compulsion is short-term and intensive (acute withdrawal) and long-term attraction (protracted withdrawal) as well as an emotional and psychological adhesiveness.

Drug Addiction as Attachment and Love

Drug Addiction and Love

Drug addiction can be regarded as a substituted attachment object for clients. In many ways, love and addiction have many similarities.

> The addict is a person who never learns to come to grip with his world, and who therefore seeks stability and reassurance through some repeated, ritualized activity. This activity is reinforced in two ways: first, by a comforting sensation of well induced by the drug or other addictive object; second, by the atrophy of the addict's other interests and abilities and the general deterioration of his situation while he is preoccupied with the addiction. As alternatives grow smaller, the addiction grows larger, until it is all there is. A true addict progresses into a monomania, whether the object of addiction is a drug or a lover. Vicky and Bruce's sheltered childhoods denied them the self-confidence and the well-formed enthusiasms that a complete life is built on. As a result, they fastened out each other as a daily habit, and this habit became the raison d'etre of their existence. (Peele 1975: 27)

Peele (1975) affirmed that in people with drug addiction, their abilities to seek pleasure in normal activities are gradually deteriorated by their drug addiction. Drugs become their lover. They are so attached to drugs as drug addiction becomes the aim of their existence.

> There is a fundamental similarity between opiate addiction and love. In both cases, a person repeatedly seeks out a kind of stimulation which in intensely pleasurable. But as time goes on, he finds that he needs it more even as he enjoys it less. The heroin addict gets less and less of a positive kick from the drug, yet he must return to it to counteract the insistent pain caused by its absence. The lover is no longer so excited by his or her partner, but is more and more dependent on the comfort of the partner's continued presence, and is less able to handle a separation. Here the negative aftereffect overcomes initially positive stimulation. (Peele 1975: 53)

In other words, people seek pleasure in drug as they do in love affairs (Peele, 1975). As the tolerance effects of drugs increases, the individual needs to increase the dosage of intake so to sustain the same degree of pleasure s/he initially has. Gradually, the individual uses the drug most of his/her time and becomes more and more dependent on it. S/he becomes more and more intolerant to the separation and absence of drugs (addictive and lovable object).

Addiction to Experience

Clients with drug addiction are addicted to experiences. The addictive experience is an involvement shield and their personal ecology. Involvement in their addictive experiences is rewarding and gratifies their unfulfilled wishes as well as covers up their negative emotions, such as fear, inferiority, loneliness, anger, and emptiness. Gradually, their involvement in addictive experiences becomes their daily pattern with severe disturbance to their normal daily life.

> Because addiction is finally a human phenomenon, it engages every aspect of a person's functioning, starting with the rewards (as interpreted by the individual) that an involvement provides and the individual's need for these rewards. The motivation to pursue the involvement, as compared with other alternatives, is a function of an additional layer of social, situational and personality variables.... (Peele 1985: 97)

Peele (1985) affirmed that different types of addictive experiences from drugs match with various kinds of unfulfilled addictive needs according to the client's own unique beliefs in power, controllability, and legal and moral interpretation of related experiences. Addictive needs are reflected in related social milieu, individual traits, and needs as well as an individual's values and needs. Peele (1985) affirmed that addictive needs are related to personal, interpersonal, and social variables. Addictive experiences and needs interact with one another, making the individual fully engage or attach to drug addiction.

Addiction and Attachment

People with insecure attachment always embrace intense negative emotions, such as anger and fear of being abandoned by others. Furthermore, they also have fear of intimacy in relating to others (Bowen 1976, 1978; Hazen and Shaver 1987). All these negative emotions make them become vulnerable in using addictive experiences as substituted attachment (Cooper et al. 1998; Dottan et al. 2003). Hoefler and Kooyman (1996) affirmed that drug addiction is a delayed maladaptive attachment transition in young adults with an associated fear of intimacy. Similarly, Descutner and Thelen (1991) asserted that the fear of intimacy is a risk factor for emotional problems and substance abuse. Finally, Thorberg and Lyvers (2006) found out that subjects with drug addiction embrace higher levels of insecure attachment and fear of intimacy. They have lower levels of secure attachment and differentiation of self in comparison with those in control groups (Thorberg and Lyvers 2006: 723).

A Holistic Human Dimension of Drug Addiction

Drug addiction interacts with various dimensions of the client, including his/her meaning of life, self-system, mind, body, and social functioning. Each of above-mentioned concepts focuses on one dimension of a human being. It can be illustrated in the following Table 1.

Table 1. Different Dimensions of a Person and Drug Addiction and Related Perspectives (Yip 2015)

Related Dimensions in Human Beings	Related Figures and Scholars
Existential Dimension: Meaning of Life	The choice of drug addiction is a way to ease out of their pain, anxiety, meaninglessness, and frustration in life (Wurm 2003)
Self-System (Self-Identity, Self-Image, and Self-Boundary)	Narcissus' model in interpretation of addiction and treatment Khantzian (1980, 1981) based on self-pathology, asserted substance abuse, and drug addiction is actually a matter of self-choice. Different persons because of various types of personalities and unfulfilled psychological needs generated from self-pathology, they tend to choose their own types of drugs.
Mind: Cognition	Cognitive harm reduction approach
Mind: Emotion	Khantizian model, Peele model, Wurmser model, and Khantzian model also concern of emotions.
Mind: Experiences and Memories	Peel's addiction to experience
Body	Pharmacological harm reduction approach Physiological effects of different kinds of drugs
Behaviors: Social Functioning, Roles, and Interpersonal Relationships	Wurmser (1978) affirmed that drug addiction and substance abuse is, in fact, a kind of compulsiveness Attachment and drug addiction Love and addiction

Each of the above-mentioned perspectives may imply focusing on one human dimension. Additionally, there are three foci among all these perspectives.

1. Focus on deficit and destructive power of drug addiction (e.g., harm reduction approach).

2. Focus on unfulfilled need of any one dimension of the human being that needs to be pathologically coped with drug addiction and substance abuse.
3. Focus on addiction of drug-induced experiences, stimulated physiological and psychological effects rather than the drug itself (Yip 2015).

Thus, to have a holistic, humanistic, and multi-dimensional understanding of clients with drug addiction and abuse, different human dimensions, including, body, emotionality, stress and coping, attachment, self-system, and the meaning of life should be included in interpretation and intervention for clients with drug addiction.

NATURES AND DESTRUCTIVE EFFECTS OF TRAUMA

Traumatic Event Defined in DSM IV

Traumas include a wide range of natural disasters, interpersonal oppression and abuse that create a seriously destructive effect on their victims physically and mentally. There are many definitions of traumas. In DSM IV, traumatic events are defined as follows:

> Traumatic events that are experienced directly include, but are not limited to military combat, violent personal assault (sex assault, physical attack, robbery, mugging, being kidnapped, being taken hostage, terrorist attack, torture, incarceration as a prisoner of war or in a concentration camp, natural or manmade disasters, severe automobile accidents or being diagnosed with a life-threatening illness.
>
> For children, sexually traumatic events may include developmentally inappropriate sexual experiences without threatened or actual violence or injury.
>
> Witnessed events include, but are not limited to, observing the serious injury or unnatural death of another person due to violent assault, serious accident, or disaster or unexpectedly witnessing a dead body or body parts.

Events experienced by others that are learned about include, but are not limited to, violent personal assault, serious accident, or serious injury experienced by a family member or a close friend, or learning about a sudden, unexpected death of a family member or a close friend, or learning that one's child has a life-threatening disease.

The trauma is especially serious and long lasting if the trauma is induced by others (torture, rape).

Re-experiencing of the traumatic event may be in forms of dreams, intrusive recollection, or dissociative flashback in seconds or even in hours. (American Psychiatric Association 1994: 443)

From DSM IV definition, the following natures are described:

A: People involved in Traumatic Event
A1: The Victim of the Trauma
A2: The Witness of the Trauma
A3: Victims' Significant Others Learn about the Trauma

B: Related Traumas Events
B1: Accidents
B2: Natural Disaster
B2: Warfare
B3: Personal Violence
(Physical Attack, Sex Assaults, Being Kidnapped)
B4: News about Terminal Illness

C: Duration of Traumas
C1: Short
C2: Long Lasting

D: Effects of Trauma
D1: Immediate Effect during the Traumas
D2: Rebound nd Recall of Trauma
D3: Chronic Effect of Trauma

Acute Stress Disorder and Post-traumatic Stress Disorder

The destructive effects of traumas have three types:
D1: Immediate effect during the traumas
D2: Re-bounce and recall of trauma
D3: Chronic effect of trauma

The immediate destructive effects of trauma are described as "acute stress disorder" in DSM IV. The rebounce and recall of trauma is named "post-traumatic stress disorder" (PTSD).

Acute Stress Disorder: Diagnosis, Symptoms and Etiology

The symptoms of acute stress disorder are described in DSM IV as follows:

A. the person has been exposed to a traumatic event in which both of the following were present:
    1) a subjective sense of numbing, detachment, or absence of emotional responsiveness.
    2) a reduction in awareness of his or her surroundings (e.g., being in a daze)
    3) derealization
    4) depersonalization
    5) dissociative amnesia (i.e., inability to recall an important aspects of the trauma)
B. Either while experiencing or after experiencing the distressing event, the individual has three (or more) of the following dissociative symptoms: recurrent image, thoughts, dreams, illusion
C. The traumatic event is persistently reexperienced in at least one of the following: recurrent images, thoughts, dreams, illusions, flashback episode, or a sense of relieving the experience, or distress on exposure to remember of the traumatic event.

D. Marked avoidance of stimuli that arouse recollections of the trauma (e.g., thoughts, feelings, conversations, activities, places, people).
E. Marked symptoms of anxiety or increased arousal (e.g., difficulty sleeping, irritability, poor concentration, hypervigilance, exaggerated startle response, motor resilience).
F. The disturbance causes clinically significant distress or impairment in social, occupational, or other important areas of functioning or impairs the individual's ability to pursuer some necessary task, such as obtaining necessary assistance or mobilizing personal resources by telling family members about the traumatic experience.
G. The disturbance lasts for a minimum of 3 days and a maximum of 4 weeks of the traumatic events
H. The disturbance is not due to the direct physiological effects of a substance (e.g., a drug of abuse, a medication) or a general medical condition, is not better accounted for by brief psychotic disorder, and is not merely an exacerbation of a pre-existing Axis I or Axis II disorder.

(American Psychiatric Association 1994: 324)

Associated features:

1) symptoms of despair and hopelessness may be experiences in Acute stress disorder and may be sufficiently severe and persistent to meet criteria of major depressive disorder.
2) survivors of the trauma may have strong sense of guilt of another's death that leads to ignore of health and basic safety after the trauma. Impulsive and risk-taking behavior may occur after the trauma.

Culture Features:

Many symptoms and response to trauma may be culturally bounded and defined.

Prevalence

It all depends on the severity and persistence of the trauma.

Course:

1) symptoms occur immediately during after the trauma, last for at least two days, and either resolve within 4 weeks after the conclusion of the traumatic event or the diagnosis is changed.
2) When symptoms persist beyond 1 month, a diagnosis of post-traumatic stress disorder may be appropriate
3) the severity, duration, and proximity of an individual's exposure to the trauma tend to the most important factors in determining the likelihood of the development of this disorder

(American Psychiatric Association 1994: 324)

From the above-mentioned description, it is clear acute stress disorder is actually a numbing toward traumatic experiences in which the individual tries to survive within the trauma.

According to Yip (2013), the numbing is a kind of self-dissociation from traumatic experiences. According to the above-mentioned diagnosis, the numbing in traumatic experiences manifests in the following ways:

1) *numbing of client's sense of mind* (difficulties in concentration, avoiding of recollection of memory in trauma). It is also a retardation of individual's cognitive processing of related message, image and information in the traumatic experiences
2) *numbing of client's sense of self* (dissociative amnesia, sometimes including self identity, intensive of sense of depersonalization—loss of the sense of being a lively person)
3) *numbing of client's sense of environment* (severe sense of derealization, reduction of awareness to environment including time, space, color and brightness). It is a retardation of related perception and reception of the fear from the traumatic and life-threatening environment
4) *numbing of client's sense of body* (retarded sense of pain and hurt and increase toleration of wound and hurt)
5) *numbing of client's sense of growth* (fixation on traumatic experience and inability to grow and develop). It is also a

> retardation of one's ability to predict the future within traumatic experiences. (Yip 2013)

The numbing of five senses in the self-dissociation mechanism means that the individual's detective, receptive, and processing power within the traumatic experiences are greatly slowed down or even paralyzed so that the destructive effects toward the self-system, mind, and body are immediately reduced. In an extreme situation, the individual does not feel pain and fear. The fight-or-flight mechanism in avoiding fearful stimuli is replaced by a high-tolerance mechanism. It allows the individual to retain his/her minimal physical functioning so as to survive within traumatically fearful experiences. Within dissociative traumatic fear, the fearful senses are numbed, temporarily retarded, but not permanently impaired. Intensive fear still penetrates into the mind, the self-system, and the memories of the individual, but it is temporarily stored, suppressed, and repressed. However, the numbing not only retard one's five senses in inhibiting the destructive effect or intensive fear and threat from environment, it also temporarily retards the ego and social functioning of the individual. Immediately after the traumatic experience, the individual appears to be numbed and dissociated for a period of time without expression of intensive fear or traumatic suffering. That means, the individual still inhibits part of his/her ego and social functioning so as to save and ensure the integrity of the ego and self-system (Yip 2013).

Post-Traumatic Stress Disorder, Diagnosis, Symptoms, and Etiology

As the individual ego and social functioning return to normal, the stored, suppressed, or repressed traumatic dissociative fear rebounds. The reassociation of repressed and dissociative traumatic fear implies that the mind, self-system, and the body of the individual prepares to resolve and integrate the traumatic dissociative fear. The more traumatic the experience is, the more powerful the rebound of the traumatic fear. In psychopathological terms, it is the PTSD symptoms (Yip 2013). According to DSM IV, they are listed as follows:

A. person has been exposed to a traumatic event in which both the following were present:
   1) the person experienced, witnessed, or was controlled with an event or events that involved actual or threatened death or serious injury, or a threat to the physical integrity of self or others.
   2) the person's response involved intense fear, helplessness, or horror.

(Note: in children, this may be expressed instead by disorganized of agitated behavior)

B. the traumatic event is persistently re-experienced in one or more of the following ways:
   1) recurrent and intrusive distressing recollection of the event, including images, thoughts or perceptions. Note: in young children, repetitive play may occur in which themes or aspects of the trauma are expected.
   2) recurrent distressing dreams of the events. Note: in children, here may be frightening dreams without recognizable content.
   3) acting or feeling as if the traumatic event were recurring (includes a sense of reliving the experience, illusions, hallucinations, and dissociative flashback episodes, including those that occur on awakening or when intoxicated) Note: in young children, trauma-specific reenactment may occur.
   4) intense psychological distress at exposure to internal or external cues that symbolize or resemble an aspect of the traumatic events.
   5) physiological reactivity on exposure to internal or external cues that symbolize or resemble an aspect of the traumatic events.
C. Persistent avoidance of stimuli associated with the trauma and numbing of general responsiveness (nor present before the trauma) as indicated by three or more of the following:

1) efforts to avoid thoughts, feelings or conversations associated with the trauma.
2) efforts to avoid activities, places or people that arouse recollections of the trauma.
3) inability to recall an important aspect of the trauma.
4) markedly diminished interest or participation in significant activities.
5) feeling of detachment or estrangement from others.
6) restricted range of affect (e.g., unable to have loving feeling).
7) sense of a foreshortened future (e.g., does not expect to have a career, marriage, children, or a normal life span).

D. Persistent symptoms of increased arousal (not present before the trauma), as indicated by two or more of the following:
1) difficulty falling or staying asleep
2) irritability or outburst of anger
3) difficulty concentrating
4) hypervigilance
5) exaggerated startle response

E. Duration of the disturbance (symptoms in criteria A, B, C and D) is more than 1 month.

F. The disturbance causes clinically significant distress or impairment in social, occupational, or other important areas of functioning.

Specific if
Acute: if duration of symptoms is less than 3 months

Chronic: if duration of symptoms is 3 months or more
Specific if

With *Delayed Onset:* if onset of symptoms is at least 3 months after the stressor (American Psychiatric Association 1994: 425–7)

From all these listed symptoms, Yip (2013) affirmed that dissociative traumatic fear together with related experiences can rebound/reassociate in various forms of:

a) *full conscious rebound*/reassociation (FCR) in forms of intrusive distressing recollection of events, including images, thoughts, and perception
b) full unconscious rebound/reassociation (FUR) in forms of distressing dream
c) *partial conscious rebound*/reassociation (PCR) in forms of flashback, illusion, hallucinations and related episodes
d) *partial unconscious rebound*/reassociation (PUR) in forms of psychological and/or psychological distress being triggered by external and internal clues that symbolize or resemble an aspect of the traumatic events

All these represent various degrees of rebound and reassociation of traumatic fear ranging from a full conscious rebound to a partial unconscious rebound. According to different background, resilience, and experiences, the process of rebound can exist in various combinations and ways as follows:

1. FCR then FUR then PCR and finally PUR (*Gradual decrease of power of rebound*). It can be a gradual absorption and integration of traumatic fear into the self-system (FCR, FUR, PCR, and PUR and finally resolution of traumatic fear). It can also mean the dissociation of the traumatic fear is necessary, but the dissociative effect and mechanism is not as powerful as before.
2. PUR then PCR then FUR and finally FCR (*Gradual increase of power of rebound*) Due to the increase of intensity of triggers in unpleasant immediate environment, it can be a gradual and full rebound of traumatic fear so that the individual is able to reintegrate it into the internal system (FCR, FUR, PCR, and PUR and resolution of traumatic fear). It can also be a further dissociation as the full rebound is too painful for the individual to face it.
3. FCR and/or FUR rebound (*Full conscious and unconscious rebound*). Full rebound may mean the dissociative traumatic fear accumulated is too powerful to an extent that the individual's internal system cannot absorb or dissociate anymore. Instead, it

rebounds fully, creating a prevailing recall of fearful and traumatic experiences within which the individual's ego in its daily functioning life is deeply affected. However, it also means the full rebound of traumatic fear allows the individual, with proper external support, can resolve and integrate the traumatic fear into the internal system. If the individual has a good resolution of dissociative traumatic fear, s/he can full integrate this traumatic fear into his/her own internal system (*FCR and/or FUR rebound and a full resolution*). If the individual cannot resolve it or there is further input of traumatic fear, then the individual needs to dissociate his/her former traumatic experience as well as new traumatic experience (FCR and/or FUR rebound + former and new traumatic fear and experience).

4. PCR and/or PUR rebound (*Partial conscious and unconscious rebound*) Partial rebound means related traumatic fearful experiences are still needed to be partially dissociated so as to avoid the overwhelming destructive effects imposed on the individual. Partial rebound may also mean related dissociative traumatic experiences are not intensive enough to deserve a full rebound. Within the partial rebound, if the individual has a good resolution of dissociative traumatic fear, s/he can full integrate this traumatic fear into his/her own internal system (PCR and/or PUR and a full resolution). In some cases, traumatic fear after partial rebound needs to be continuously dissociated due to personal and environmental limitations that do not allow a full rebound of traumatic fear, or the individual needs a gradual process of rebound and resolve dissociative traumatic fear.
5. FCR and/or PCR rebound (*Full and partial conscious rebound*). Full and partial conscious rebound means that the individual is fully conscious in the process of rebound. In other words, the individual's internal system can no longer suppress or repress the traumatic fear. It is out of the tolerance and dissociation limits of the individual's internal system. Within a conscious rebound, the sense of traumatic fear is clearly felt by the individual. It also allows the individual to

revisit any fine details within the process of traumatic experiences. If the individual has a good resolution of dissociative traumatic fear, s/he can full integrate this traumatic fear into his/her own internal system (FCR and/or PUR then a full resolution of traumatic fear). In some cases, the individual may not be able to have a resolution and need further dissociation of traumatic fear by avoiding related triggers (FCR and/or PUR and further dissociation).

6. FUR and/or PUC rebound (*Full and partial unconscious rebound*). Full and partial unconscious rebound means that the individual is not aware of the rebound. The rebound either appears in dreams as nightmares or as an unrecognized physiological response to external triggers. As it is unconscious and unexpected, it arouses a sort of secondary fear and anxiety for the individual. The individual may embrace a panic attack without acknowledging why and how it happens. Instead of tracing back the original traumatic experiences, the individual may regard the unconscious rebound as related to things, events, and persons (triggers) in the environment (FUR and/or PUR plus second traumatic experience). Secondary traumatic experiences may need to be further dissociated. In very mild unconscious rebound, it can be residual effects of traumatic experiences after they have resolved and integrated in the self-system (FUR and/or PUR resolved but residual effect) (Yip 2013).

The Breaking, Loss, and Repression in Trauma

Every trauma has a high destructive effect on related victims. Garland, within a psychodynamic perspective, described this destructive effect fully as follows:

> A traumatic event is one which, for a particular individual, breaks through or overrides the discriminatory, filtering process, and overrides any temporary denial or patch up of the damage.

> The mind is flooded with a kind and degree of stimulation that is far more than it can make sense of or manage. ....
>
> There is a massive disruption in functioning, amounting to a kind of breakdown. It is a breakdown of an established way of going about one's life, of established beliefs about the predictability of the world, of established mental structures, of an established defensive organization.
>
> It leaves the individual vulnerable to intensive and overwhelming anxieties form internal sources as well as from the actual external events.
>
> (Garland 1998: 10–11)

Breaking Process of Trauma

Garland's (1998) descriptions presume the breaking process of trauma as follows:

1. Flooding of external stimulation that is beyond an individual's sense or management.
2. Breaking through or overriding of the individual's discriminatory, filtering, temporary denial, and healing mechanisms.
3. The external violence in trauma penetrates and triggers inner breaking mechanisms.
4. Massive disruption of one's ego functioning, life, beliefs, mental structure, and defensive mechanism.
5. Individuals become highly vulnerable to external and internal anxiety after the breakdown of related mechanisms.

Effects of Loss in Trauma

> Loss of good object: Loss of good self, prevailing bad self and bad others, hostility toward self and others. (My life has gone to pieces; I've lost my interest and pleasure in daily life; I feel stressful and tense in doing even small things. I become angry at myself and others.)

- Traumatic breakdown of ego functioning in: filtering discriminatory process
- Denial of damage
- Loss of security and predictability of current and future life

- Confirmation of universal anxiety (Garland 1998: 11–12)

Apart from the breaking force, *the effect of loss also occurs in trauma.* The process and components of loss also include the following:

1. Loss of good object with prevailing bad other (hostility toward others)
2. Loss of good self with prevailing bad self (hostility toward self)
3. Loss of security and predictability of current and future life
4. Loss of sense of security and ability to adapt and cope with anxiety
5. Loss of inner ability to admit, to tolerate, and to heal inner wound and damage

Repression in Trauma

In addition to the effects of loss and breaking, the repression mechanism of the individual is also shattered.

> Freud death instinct and beyond pleasure principles: (breakdown of usual immoral belief in facing others' death, hostility towards self and insecurity towards life and future.)
>
> - Mourning of loss of objects in the trauma.
> - Over and prevailing negative stimuli out of the internal resources to take up and absorbed. (Garland 1998: 11–12)

The shattered effects of repression mechanism include the following:

1. Trauma is a foreign body that shatters an individual's repressive mechanism.
2. Awakening of repressed unpleasant objects, events, and memories in the past.
3. Breaking down of one's morality system and arousal of one's death instinct.

The Wounded Self

The breaking, the loss, and the shattering of the repression mechanism may finally make the victim of trauma become powerless, fragmented, disconnected, and vulnerable. Herman (1992) defined trauma as the wounding of self:

> Trauma is the wounding of self. Traumatic experiences are about being rendered utterly powerless, in the face of an atrocity (caused by another person) or a disaster (caused by nature). Traumatic events overwhelm our ability to feel a sense of control, connection and meaning….psychological trauma as a process of withdrawal and disconnection. In withdrawing from the world traumatized people lose connection to that which is meaningful…family, community, spiritual life. In addition, trauma can impair people's ability to rejuvenate and recuperate as a result, they are more susceptible to the debilitating effects of subsequent traumatic events. (Herman 1992: 33–34)

Herman (1992) affirmed the wounding effects of traumas as follows:

1. Powerlessness
2. Loss of self-control
3. Sense of disconnection and meaninglessness
4. Withdrawal
5. Vulnerable to further trauma

In the same of thinking, Carruth and Burke described the destructive effect of trauma as follows:

> Psychological trauma, in its broadest sense, is a wound to one's self, one's personhood. Trauma impacts how people perceive their worlds, their thoughts, judgments, and intuition, what feelings they allow themselves to have and what feelings they can't stop themselves from having. Perhaps most importantly, *trauma impacts people's sense of who they are as unique individuals and their sense of soul—one's connection to something greater*

> *than the self.* Trauma simultaneously causes hyper-arousal and emotional constriction. The strategies people develop to contain and manage these trauma reactions can ultimately develop into a disorder of control—being out of control and trying to be in control. (Carruth and Burke 2006: 2)

Carruth and Bruke (2006) described the wounding effects of traumas in the following details:

1) Trauma impacts one's perception on the worlds as well as their thought, judgment and intuition (Distortion of perception, thought, judgment and intuition).
2) It shakes one's self control, senses of uniqueness and ability to connect with the outside world (Distortion gradually leads to shaking one's self-system in terms of uniqueness and self-control).
3) It causes hyper-arousal and emotional constriction in which the individual has to contain and manage these reaction (Together with the shaking of one's self-system and distortion is an absorption of emotional constriction and hyper-arousal of mind, body and self).
4) Strategies to contain, to absorb, and to manage restricted emotion and hyper-arousal will finally break down leading to disorder in the self-system.

> Traumatic events injure a person's dignity and sense of integrity. People often feel damaged, incomplete, and less human as a result of the experience. At the same time, trauma challenges and alters people's beliefs about their world, their potency, benevolence, significance and worthiness and damages their ability to trust themselves and the environment.
>
> As a result, traumatized people are often more guarded and less willing to venture out and take risks. Trauma also distorts people sense of time and timing.. (Carruth and Burke 2006: 2)

Carruth and Burke (2006) clearly describe the result of the breaking down of the self-system after the trauma. They can be listed as follows:

1. Injures of individual's dignity and integrity
2. Feeling of being incomplete and less human
3. Challenge of one's belief in human values such as benevolence, significance, potency, and worthiness
4. Damage of trust toward oneself and others
5. Increase in ego defense and self-guard in social interactions
6. Decrease in adaptation to new challenges and taking risks
7. Sense of time and sense of being are distorted and defined by traumatic events
8. Judgment and act are impaired with results of impulsivity and hesitation

A Comprehensive Process of Traumatization

The above-mentioned description can be combined as a comprehensive process of traumatization. This process should have the following components and stages:

- Natures of Trauma: people involved (A), related events (B), duration (C)
- Immediate Effects of Trauma: acute stress disorder (D)
- Prolonged Effect: Rebound and Recall of Traumatic Experiences: PTSD (Recollection) (E)
- Prolonged Effect: Avoidance and further suppression of Recall of Traumatic Experiences: PTSD (Avoidance) (F)
- Prolonged Effect: Increase of Arousal in Traumatic Disturbance: PTSD (Increase in arousal) (G)
- Chronic Effect of Trauma: Breaking Effect (H)
- Chronic Effect of Trauma: Loss Effect (I)
- Chronic Effects of Trauma: Awakening of Unpleasant Repression (J)
- Chronic Effects of Trauma: Wounded Self (K)

From DSM IV definition, the following natures are described:

A: Natures of Trauma: People involved
A1: The Victim of the Trauma
A2: The Witness of the Trauma
A3: Victims' Significant Others Learn about the Trauma

B: Natures of Trauma: Related Events
B1: Accidents
B2: Natural Disaster
B2: Warfare
B3: Personal Violence (Physical Attack, Sex Assaults, Being Kidnapped)
B4: News about Terminal Illness

C: Natures of Trauma: Duration
C1: Short
C2: Long Lasting

D: Immediate Effect during the Trauma: Acute Stress Disorder
D1: numbing of client's sense of mind (difficulties in concentration, avoiding of recollection of memory in trauma).
D2: numbing of client's sense of self (dissociative amnesia, sometimes including self-identity, intensive of sense of depersonalization—loss of the sense of being a lively person)
D3: numbing of client's sense of environment (severe sense of derealization, reduction of awareness to environment including time, space, color and brightness).
D4: numbing of client's sense of body (retarded sense of pain and hurt and increase toleration of wound and hurt)

D5: numbing of client's sense of growth (fixation on traumatic experience and inability to grow and develop). (Yip 2013)
D6: some may harbor hopelessness and despairs
D7: survivors may harbor intensive guilt towards those died in trauma
D8: recollection of traumatic experiences within 3 days to 4 weeks

E: Rebound and recall of Traumatic Experiences: Post-traumatic Stress Disorder (Recollection)
E1: Full conscious rebounce/re-association in forms of intrusive distressing recollection of events, including images, thought and perception. (FCR)
E2: Full unconscious rebounce/re-association in forms of distressing dream. (FUR)
E3: Partial conscious rebounce/re-association in forms of flashback, illusion, hallucinations and related episodes (PCR)
E4: Partial unconscious rebounce/re-association in forms of psychological and/or psychological distress being triggered by external and internal clues that symbolize or resemble an aspect of the traumatic events (PUR) (Yip 2013)

F: Avoidance and further suppression of Recall of Traumatic Experiences: Post-Traumatic Stress Disorder (Avoidance)
F1: Specific Internal Avoidance: avoiding related thoughts, feeling or conversation associated with the trauma
F2: Specific External Avoidance: avoiding activities, place or people that arouse recollection of the trauma
F3a: General Internal Avoidance (a): Inability to recall an important event of trauma
F3b: General Internal Avoidance (b): Restricted range of affect
F4a: General External Avoidance (b): markedly diminished interest or participation in significant activities

F4b: General External Avoidance (b): Feeling of detachment or estrangement from others

F4c: General External Avoidance (c): Sense of a foreshortened future (American Psychiatric Association: 1994)

G: Increase of Arousal in Traumatic Disturbance: Post Traumatic Stress Disorder (Increase in arousal)

G1: Difficulty falling or staying asleep

G2: Irritability or outburst of anger

G3: Difficulty concentrating

G4: Hyper-vigilance

G5: Exaggerated startle response (American Psychiatric Association 1994)

H: Chronic Effect of Trauma: Breaking Effect

H1: Flooding of external stimulation that is beyond individuals' sense or management

H2: Breaking through or overriding of individuals' discriminatory, filtering, temporary denial and healing mechanisms

H3: The external violence in trauma penetrates and triggers inner breaking mechanisms

H4: Massive disruption of one's ego functioning, life, beliefs, mental structure, and defensive mechanism

H5: Individuals become highly vulnerable to external and internal anxiety after the breakdown of related mechanisms. (Garland 1998)

I: Chronic Effect of Trauma: Loss Effect

I1: Loss of good object with prevailing bad other (hostility towards others)

I2: Loss of good self with prevailing bad self (hostility towards self)

I3: Loss security and predictability of current and future life
I4: Loss of sense of security and ability to adapt and cope with anxiety
I5: Loss of inner ability to admit, to tolerate and to heal inner wound and damage

J: Chronic Effects of Trauma: Awakening of Unpleasant Repression
J1: Shattering the repressive mechanism
J2: Awakening of repressed unpleasant object, event and memories in the past
J3: Awakening of anger and hate towards uncaring significant others including parents, siblings, colleagues, teachers and friends
J4: Awakening of death instinct and beyond pleasure principles
J5: Awakening of hostility towards self and others
J6: Awakening of insecurity towards life and future

K: Chronic Effects of Trauma: Wounded Self
K1: Sense of powerlessness
K2: Loss of self uniqueness and self control
K3: Sense of disconnection and meaninglessness
K4: Withdrawal (Herman 1992)
K5: Injuries of one's dignity and integrity
K6: Feeling of incomplete and less humane
K7: Challenge of one's belief in human values such as benevolence, significance, potency and worthiness
K8: Damage of trust towards oneself and others
K9: Increase in ego defense and self guard in social interaction
K10: Decrease in adaptation to new challenges and take risks
K11: Sense of time and sense of being are distorted and defined by traumatic events
K12: Judgment and act is impaired with results of impulsivity and hesitation.
Carruth and Bruke (2006)

All these are illustrated in the following figure 1.

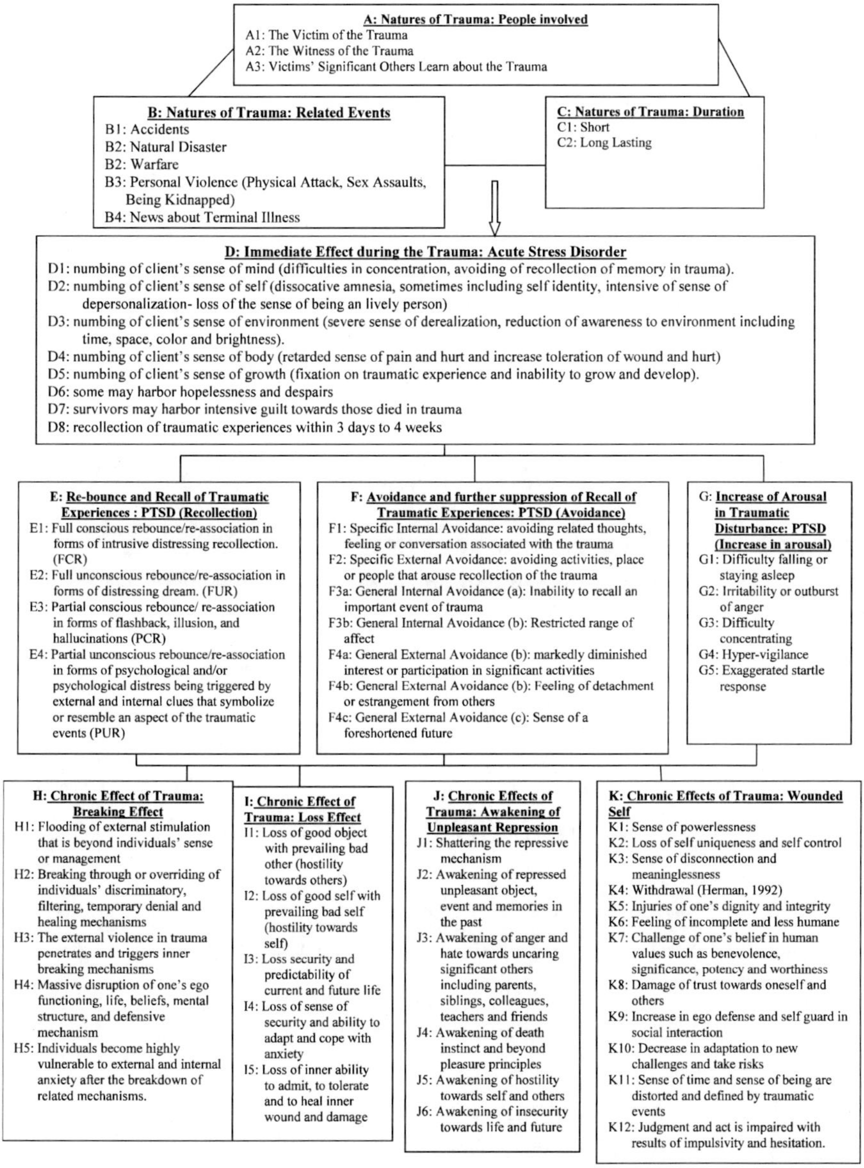

Figure 1. The Natures and Destructive Effects of Trauma.

Trauma and Mental Illness

From the above-mentioned discussion, it is clear that acute effects, rebound, and recall effects as well as the chronic effects of trauma all have close relationships with the onset of various types of mental illness.

Acute Effect = Acute Stress Disorder and Dissociative Disorder
Recall, Avoidance, and Arousal of Disturbance = Post-Traumatic Stress Disorder
Chronic Effects: the Loss Effect = Depression and Major Depressive Disorder
Chronic Effects: the Breaking Effect = Schizophrenia and Dissociative Disorder
Chronic Effects: the Awakening Effect = Anxiety Disorders
Chronic Effects: the Wounded Self = Personality Disorder

In the acute effects of traumatic events, the individual suffers from severe numbing of body and mind. Prolonged numbing may result in a dissociative disorder, as the individual needs to suppress and repress related traumatic experiences to avoid retraumatization. For PTSD, there are three main groups of symptoms: recall, avoidance, stimuli arousal.

The recall effect is actually the rebound of the suppressed traumatic experiences. There is partial or full rebound as well as conscious or unconscious rebound. Individuals with severe traumatic experiences may first have full conscious rebound and gradually decrease to partial conscious rebound and then to partial unconscious rebound. For many individuals with severe traumatic experiences, their rebound may continue and last for their whole lives. Their rebound may not be full or conscious; however, they will still have the occasional full conscious rebound, such as having distressing dreams at night. Some may suffer from unconscious partial rebound with unpleasant triggering from external stimuli. In a normal case, the recall effect in PTSD implies that the self-system of the individual gradually absorbs the suppressed and repressed traumatic experiences and memories. Thus, with persistent and good support from significant others, the full conscious rebound from the victims of trauma may slowly or gradually turn into partial or unconscious rebound and finally become resolved. However, for those repeated traumas, or the individuals with poor mental or physical conditions that are vulnerable to trauma, these recall effects may persist for a long time or may even be a lifelong process, making the individual highly vulnerable to stress with spontaneous symptoms of depressive mood, anxiety, or psychosomatic symptoms.

The avoidance symptoms imply specific internal and external avoidance in which the individual consciously avoids related thoughts, feelings, and conversation or/and avoids activities, places, or people related with the trauma. Also, there are general internal and external avoidance in which the individual is unable to recall important events of trauma, restricted affect, marked diminishing interest or participating in significant activities, feeling of detachment, or a loss of hope. In PTSD, the avoidance effect is actually an inner mechanism to protect the individual from reexperiencing the pain in trauma (retraumatization). However, it also means that the self-system and mind of the trauma victim fail or is not ready to resolve the traumatic experiences.

In normal cases, the avoidance mechanism may last for a period of time. After the recollection of traumas and the appropriate healing process, the avoidance mechanism may gradually decrease as time goes by. If the avoidance mechanism lasts for a long time, it may be because the destructive impacts of the traumas are too strong and the individual needs a very long time to absorb it before starting the self-healing recollection process. It may also be due to repeated traumas or regular retraumatization, such as repeated physical abuse by significant others. The avoidance and suppression mechanisms are the only way for the individual to take a rest from all these destructive effects of the traumas. In some extreme cases, the avoidance mechanism may persist for many years or even for a whole life in which the individual's ego functioning, social functioning, and daily life is deeply affected. For example, a client with a trauma of drowning in a swimming pool may for his or her whole life avoid approaching a swimming pool. In that sense, the avoidance symptoms for a prolonged period of time can be transformed into various kinds of phobias. Prolonged internal and external avoidance implies that the individual suffers from chronic dissociation in mind and body. As a consequence, many clients with traumatic experiences may finally end up with various forms of hysterical symptoms.

Apart from recollection and avoidance, there are also symptoms of an increase of arousal in PTSD. They manifest in forms of difficulty in falling or staying asleep, irritability or outbursts of anger, difficulty in concentration, hypervigilance, and exaggerated startle responses. It implies that the individual is still on a highly alert mental and physical condition as they are facing or experiencing highly risky and traumatic situations. In doing so, their mental and physical energy is deeply consumed. Because of consuming inner psychic energy in avoidance (suppression) as well as rebound and resolution (recollection) of traumatic experiences and memories, individuals may face an adverse consequence that their inner psychic energy may finally be exhausted. That means, apart from arousal in traumatic disturbance, the individual is unable to perform his/her normal social functioning. They have poor performance in work, family, and normal social and recreational activities. Prolonged arousal in traumatic disturbance may even result in psychosomatic symptoms and anxiety disorders.

In effect, the three major groups of symptoms—recollection effects, avoidance effects, and arousal effects—are closely related to one another. While the recollection effects are a rebound of the traumatic memories, avoidance is a conscious way to avoid all of this. However, the arousal effect implies that even though the individual tries to avoid and even suppress or repress it, the mind still has its own limitations. If the traumatic experiences are too strong, durable, and intensive, the individual may not have enough psychic power to suppress all these strong traumatic memories. Even the traumatic experiences have been intensively recollected for some time, and the individual tries by all means to avoid being triggered. However, the residual destructive effects of the traumatic experiences are still there in which the individual requires extra energy to suppress their normal daily social and ego functioning. In doing so, his/her ego energy is being greatly reduced, in which the unconscious partial arousal of suppressed traumatic experiences in forms of insomnia, outbursts of anger, difficulty in concentration, hypervigilance, and exaggerated startle responses are common.

In fact, these three groups of symptoms—recollection, avoidance, arousal—may have different manifestations in different types and negative impacts of traumas. For those single-incident-based traumatic accidents or disasters, as the experiences are highly traumatic and disastrous, the recollection, avoidance, and arousal effects should be very intensive for a long period of time. However, for those repeated and frequent interpersonal traumas without physical abuse, such as bullying, verbal aggression, and humiliation, their recollection effects as well as the avoidance effects are highly suppressed. Any time the individual tries to recollect the traumatic memories, new repeated regular traumatic experiences come in. Furthermore, in no way can the individual avoid all these regular inputs of traumatic experiences. Thus, for repeated interpersonal traumas in life, the recollection effects and the avoidance are severely suppressed. Instead, the arousal effects may be highly intensified in forms of prolonged insomnia, great difficulty in concentration, instability, and high irritability to external responses. For traumas in physical abuse natures, if they are performed by strangers and it hurts the victims seriously, such as rape, homicide, or being kidnapped and beaten by others, the disastrous effects of the trauma is very powerful. Its recollection effects will be very severe. The individual will be deeply disturbed by the ongoing rebound of traumatic memories (related images, voices, smell, and sensations). However, if the physical abuse is done by the victim's significant others in repeated sequences, it is certain that recollection effects and avoidance effects are being suppressed. Instead, the arousal effects are very powerful. Many people with repeated traumas of physical abuse are highly sensitive to others' touch on their body. They may try by all means to avoid being touched by others. Even a slight touching may trigger their suppressed traumatic memories in an unconscious way. They simply feel uncomfortable, but they fail to link this touch to former memories of physical abuse.

In fact, different types of symptoms in PTSD may mean different types of mental illness. Recollection may imply the continuation of PTSD. Prolonged avoidance disorder may nurture a phobic disorder in which the individual tries his/her best to avoid objects, context, persons, and issues that trigger his/her recollection of traumatic memories. For prolonged arousal effects, the individual may suffer from different types of dissociative disorders in which the individual tries to paralyze part of his/her body and/or mind so as to suppress the rebound of traumatic memories.

Related chronic effects may also contribute to different types of mental problems. The breaking effects of trauma tends to shatter the individual's internal mechanism to cope with and heal from further traumatic wounds. It also has a massive disruption effect on one's ego functioning, beliefs, mental structure, and defensive mechanism. In extreme cases, it can lead to self-fragmentation in the form of schizophrenia. That is a fracturing of the ego system because of it is no longer strong enough to settle the conflict between the id and superego. It also stirs up or reactivates settled conflicts and splitting between past and present, ideal and current situation, desires and social expectation, others' perceptions, and self-identity with a resulting formation of conflicting delusions and hallucinations in his/her psychotic inner world. When the breaking effect turns into a powerful self-fragmentation, individuals do not have reasonable or good contact of the reality. Instead, s/he may be totally absorbed in his/her hallucinated and delusive self-constructed reality within which the traumatic memories, images, voices, and smells in different life stages may transform into the content of highly symbolic delusions and hallucinations.

Apart from the breaking effect, severe and prolonged trauma implies a traumatic loss to the individual. It can be a loss of part of the body or physical functioning due to physical harm in an accident or disaster. It can be a loss of family members, friends, spouses, and peers in a trauma. It can also be a loss of relationship, trust, love, and faith of significant others because of traumatic betrayal, interpersonal bullying, and oppression. After a traumatic incident, because of recollection of traumatic memories, the individual may lose his/her self-competence in facing similar situations, persons, issues, and events. The fear in facing similar situations, persons, issues, and events implies the development of various types of phobic disorders. For example, a clerk who experiences a traumatic fire in her office, after the traumatic incident, may lose his/her self-confidence in working in similar office settings. In some cases, it is also a total loss of hope in the future. It is common that a widow with three small children, whose husband was the only bread winner in the whole family, loses all her hope in the future to bring up her three children. All these losses certainly harbor various degrees of depressive moods. In severe cases, it also leads to the development of major depressive disorders.

Another chronic effect of trauma is that the individual fails to sustain his/her unpleasant repression. It usually occurs in clients facing severe traumas for the second or more time. In the first time, the individual may possess the ability either to suppress traumatic memories and experiences or to heal related wounds in traumas. However, for the second time, as his/her ego system is much more vulnerable and his/her psychic energy has been largely consumed, the individual may not able to suppress or repress the coming traumas. Instead, the traumatic memories and experiences bounce back easily. The shattering of the repressive mechanism is an awakening of repressed unpleasant object, event, and memories in the past. It is also an awakening of anger and hate toward uncaring significant others. Finally, it is an awakening of the death instinct, hostility toward self and others, as well as a sense of insecurity toward life and others. The sense of insecurity and hostility toward self and others certainly induces different types of anxiety disorders, in particular generalized anxiety disorder (GAD). The arousal of fear of similar objects, issues, contexts, and persons, as those occur in traumatic memories and experiences, may also nurture various types of phobic disorders. For example, the arousal of fear of dogs because of being bitten by a dog may cause the individual to have phobia toward dogs. The arousal of fear and anger as well as a sense of insecurity may be the major cause of personality disorders, such as antisocial personality disorder or BPD, in particular in abandonment trauma. In some cases, the spontaneous arousal of fearful memories, if being generalized in daily life or certain social context, may lead to the formation of a delusional disorder. Sometimes individuals may need to engage in chronic alcoholic abuse, drug addiction, and substance abuse to lessen the triggering and awakening effects in repressed traumatic memories.

The final chronic effect of trauma should the wounded self. That means, the destructive effects weaken the overall functioning of the whole self-system. Instead of being competent, the individual, after the trauma, becomes incompetent in daily functioning. His/her senses of uniqueness, integrity, self-control, and worth are all reduced. The more severe the chronic effects of the traumas are, the more the self-system is being destructed. As a consequence, individuals become more and more vulnerable to stress, challenges, and difficulties. Before the traumatic experiences, s/he may have been very competent in dealing with difficulties and frustrations in family, work, and other contexts in life. However, after the traumatic experiences, his/her competence in dealing similar challenges may become much less. Even very slight and mild stress, tension, and frustration may result in the formation or development of various types of mental problems. For example, a client who suffers from the traumatic loss of his left leg and right arm in a traffic accident may become highly vulnerable to stress and difficulties in a normal life pattern. Before the accident, he was a very competence chief executive officer in a large international company. However, after the accident, he does not only lose his leg and arm, but also loses his competence to be the chief executive officer in this company. The company invites him to resume his former position, but he does not feel that he can take it up again. Even worse, in the past, he could face others' negative comments in an easy and relaxed manner. Now, even a slight negative comment or label from a stranger teasing him as a crippled man makes him feel highly distressed and depressed enough to consider suicide. In everyday life, he feels anxious, depressed, and his heart breaks because he misses a good arm and leg to tackle basic social functioning.

Apart from the traumatic effects of loss, the breaking effect, the awakening effect, and the wounded self, in many cases, the dissociative or the repressive effects in PTSD still continues to make the individual highly repressive and dissociative in his ego functioning and social functioning. In some cases, the individual even has a severe dissociative disorder, such as suffering from an eating disorder, hysteria, or amnesia because of severe repression and suppression of traumatic memories and experiences.

Different Types of Traumas and Their Destructive Effects

Abandonment Trauma

There are different types of traumas before the after chronic drug addiction. Before the drug addiction, many clients encounter many life traumas, such as abandonment, abuse, bullying, and oppression by others in their childhood, adolescence, or adulthood. The destructive effects are particularly strong in childhood. Traumas suffered in childhood may mean a severe destructive effect is one's whole life.

Abandonment implies that they are being abandoned by their parents, spouses, or other significant others. Facing abandonment traumas, clients' normal developmental attachment needs are not fulfilled. They usually harbor a strong attachment hunger on one hand and have repressed abandonment fear and anger on the other hand (Yip 2013). Thus, they normally have to attach to substituted attachment figures to fulfill their attachment hunger. However, the more they attach to substituted attachment figures, the more that their abandonment fear and anger are provoked. In that case, they embrace an intimate crisis in facing their substituted attachment figures. As a consequence, they engage in endless unstable interpersonal relationships with others. On one hand, they get close to others. On the other hand, they become highly irritated by others' mild criticism and comments. Together with unstable interpersonal relationships are also unstable self-identity and unstable or even highly impulsive moods and emotions with frequent outbursts of anger and fear. Facing all these instabilities, drug addiction seems to be an instant and effective way to paralyze their unstable emotions and ambivalent relationships with others. Similar to abandonment trauma, emotional neglect and psychological abuse also has a prolonged harmful effect in childhood in one's life.

Emotional Neglect and Psychological Abuse

Emotional Neglect is defined as:

> Act of omission, frequently the result of parental ignorance or indifference. As a result, the child is not given positive emotional support and stimulation. Parents may give adequate physical care to their child but

> leave him/her alone in a crib for long period of time, seldom cuddle or talk to the child, or fail to give him/her encouragement and recognition. (Briere 1992: 8)

Furthermore, many persons with chronic drug addiction may also embrace psychological abuse by their family members or significant others in their infancy, childhood, and adolescence. It is clear that psychological abuse creates a strong destructive effect on the well-being of affected children and their development in later life. The National Center on Child Abuse and Neglect (1988) in the United States had conducted a National Study of Incidence and Severity of Child Abuse and Neglect: 200,000 cases of unambiguous emotional maltreatment occurred in United States. In this study, psychological abuse is defined in terms of eight types of parent or caretakers' behaviors:

1) Rejecting: The child is avoided or pushed away, s/he is made to feel unworthy, unacceptable and the like.
2) Degrading/devaluating: The child is criticized, stigmatized, deprived of dignity, humiliated, made to feel inferior and so on.
3) Terrorizing: The child is verbally assaulted, frightened, threatened with physical or psychological harm.
4) Isolating: The child is deprived of social contacts beyond the family, not allow friends, kept in a limited areas for long periods of time without social interaction.
5) Corrupting: The child is socialized and taught to behave in an antisocial manner, encouraged to develop socially unacceptable interests and appetites.
6) Exploiting: The child is taken advantage of, used to meet the needs of his/her caretaker.
7) Denying essential stimulation, emotional responsiveness or availability: The child is deprived of loving, sensitive caregiving: his/her emotional and intellectual development is stifled, the child is generally ignored or neglected.

8) Unreliable and inconsistent parenting: Contradictory and ambivalent demand are made of the child, parental support or caregiving is inconsistent and unreliable, and familial stability is denied the child. (Briere 1992: 9–10)

Physical Abuse

For physical abuse, it certainly including various type of physical punishments ranging from physical hitting to apathetic burning or drowning. The (National Society for Prevention of Cruelty to Children) NSPCC define physical abuse as follows:

> Physical abuse may involve hitting, shaking, throwing, poisoning, burning or scalding, drowning, suffocating, or otherwise causing physical harm to a child. Physical harm may also be caused when a parent or carer fabricates the symptoms of, or deliberately induces, illness in a child. (NSPCC 2010)

Love and Respect Organization define physical abuse in terms of the following:

> Physical abuse is any intentional and unwanted contact with you or something close to your body. Sometimes abusive behavior does not cause pain or even leave a bruise, but it's still unhealthy. Examples of physical abuse are:

- Scratching, punching, biting, strangling or kicking.
- Throwing something at you such as a phone, book, shoe or plate.
- Pulling your hair.
- Pushing or pulling you.
- Grabbing your clothing.
- Using a gun, knife, box cutter, bat, mace or other weapon.
- Smacking your bottom.
- Forcing you to have sex or perform a sexual act.

- Grabbing your face to make you look at them.
- Grabbing you to prevent you from leaving or to force you to go somewhere (Love and Respect Organization 2012).

Sex Abuse

Among various types of physical abuse, the most harmful one is sex abuse, in particular those imposed by significant others. Briere (1992) further affirmed that sex abuse has imposed a greater trauma with the following features:

Sex Abuse imposed greater trauma with the following features:

- Greater duration and frequency of the abuse
- Multiple perpetrators
- Presence of penetration or intercourse
- Physical forces sexual contact
- Abuse at an earlier age
- Molestation by a perpetrator substantially older than the victim
- Concurrent physical abuse
- Abuse involving more bizarre features
- The victim's immediate sense of personal responsibility for the molestation
- Victim feeling of powerlessness, betrayal, and/or stigma at the time of the abuse (Briere 1992: 9)

Destructive Effects of Child Abuse

The destructive effect of child abuse is severe and long lasting. It consists of three main stages.

The first stage is the initial reaction to victimization. The second stage is accommodation to ongoing abuse. The third stage is long-term elaboration and secondary accommodation.

Three Stages of impacts of Child Abuse:

1) Initial reactions to victimization: Involving post-traumatic stress, alteration in childhood development, painful affect, and cognitive distortion
2) Accommodation to ongoing abuse, involving coping behaviors intended to increase safety and/or decrease pain during victimization
3) Long-term elaboration and secondary accommodation, reflecting a): the impacts of initial reaction and abuse-related accommodations on the individual's later psychological development and b): the survivor's ongoing coping responses to abuse-related dysphoria. (Briere 1992: 17–18)

Finally, the long-term effects of child abuse should the formation of various types of pathological mental process, including the formation of possible mental illness.

Long-term Impact of Child Abuse:

1) Post-traumatic stress (re-experienced traumatic experiences such as nightmares, flashback, numbing of external response, startle response and poor concentration)
2) Cognitive distortion (dysfunctional attributions, distorted self-perception, overestimation of adversity in life, underestimation of self-efficacy and self-worth)
3) Altered emotionality (learned helplessness, powerlessness, hopelessness to deal with real, potential, or imagined threats; prolonged depression and anxiety)
4) Dissociation (disturbance or alteration of normal integrative function of identity, memory or consciousness. Sense of reality is lost and replaced by a feeling of unreality)
   a) Functions of dissociation: escape from constraints of reality; containment of traumatic memories and affects outside of normal conscious awareness; alteration or detachment of sense of self; Analgesia of pain
   b) Forms: Disengagement, dissociative disorders such as identity disorder, multiple personality and hysterical disorder
5) Impaired self-reference

6) Disturbed relatedness
7) Avoidance (Briere 1992: 17–18)

Drug Addiction and Mental Illness

Drug Addiction and Mental Illness: Causes and Effects and Different Positions

Prolonged drug addiction has a high co-morbidity with different types of mental illness. Conceptually, there may be three different types of positions regarding the relationship between mental illness and drug addiction. They are listed as follows:

1. Prolonged drug addiction leads to various types of mental illnesses.
2. Mental illness or problems are coped with and delayed by spontaneous drug addiction.
3. Drug addiction goes together with various types of mental illnesses or problems.

Regarding position number one—drug addiction leads to various types of mental illnesses—there can be three different types of causes.

1A. Prolonged drug addiction creates irreversible harm to the central nervous system, leading to mental confusion and occurrence of different types of mental illnesses, in particular schizophrenia.

1B. Prolonged drug addiction nurtures drug-related interpersonal and psychosocial traumas that lead to occurrence of different types of mental illnesses, in particular depression, BPD, and schizophrenia.

1C. Prolonged drug addiction creates irreversible harm to organs such as the liver, bladder, and kidneys. Deterioration and failure of organs nurture mental stress to the individual with a result of mental problems.

Regarding position number two—mental illnesses or mental problems are coped with and delayed by drug addiction—it can be done in several ways.

2A. Drug addiction enables the individual to escape from the painfully oppressive reality, thus delayed mental illnesses nurtures by oppressive reality.

2B. Drug addiction provides the individual a means to suppress and repress the recall and rebound of various kinds of traumas that provoked various types of mental illnesses or mental problems.

2C. Drug addiction alters the state of mind and body of the individual. At the same time, it also alters the individual's psychosocial and physical condition that leads to certain types of mental illnesses or mental problems.

Regarding position number three—drug addiction goes together with various types of mental illness or mental problems—it can also happen in several ways.

3A. Mental illnesses or problems occur before the intake of drug (mixing with the withdrawal effects of drugs).

3B. Mental illnesses or problems occur during the intake of drugs (co-morbid with the stimulating effects of drug).

3C. Mental illnesses or problems occur immediately after the intake the drug (co-morbid with after the diminishing of the stimulating effects of drugs).

3D. Mental illness or problems occur long after the intake of the drug.

Types of Drugs and Types of Mental Illness

Different types of drugs may lead to different types of mental illness because of the above-mentioned positions. However, as the trend of drug addiction and substance abuse changes drastically among drug users, the results of valid research and scholastic discussion may not be able to catch up with the trend of popular drugs among users. The most well-discussed studies of drug addiction and mental illness only occur in alcohol, amphetamines, heroine, and other common drugs. Commonly occurring mental illness in drug users are psychosis, depression, BPD, and neurosis. Most of them are empirical or small-scale studies among users in drug rehabilitation services. As they are not large-scale prevalence studies, the correlation of drug addiction can thus be only explained qualitatively rather than qualitatively. Large-scale prevalence studies can only show the prevalence of different types of mental illness including substance abuse. For example, Kilpatrick et al. (2003) implemented a national household probability sample of 4,023 telephone-interviewed adolescents ages twelve to seventeen on existing symptoms with PTSD, major depressive episodes, and substance abuse/dependence. The results showed that there are roughly 16% of boys and 19% of girls who met the criteria for at least one diagnosis. The six-month PTSD prevalence was 3.7% for boys and 6.3% for girls. The six-month major depressive episode was 7.4% for boys and 13.9% for girls. The twelve-month substance abuse/dependence prevalence was 8.2% for boys and 6.2% for girls. PTSD was more likely to be co-morbid than were major depressive episodes than substance abuse/dependence. In other words, it seems that people with drug addiction, as mentioned above, have a close relationship with related traumas. As this is only a quantitative study, the authors could not explain the refined and comprehensive relationship between trauma and drug addiction.

Drug Addiction and Psychosis/Schizophrenia

This is the most commonly observed and studied area in drug addiction and mental illness. Scholastically, it is termed as a dual diagnosis, implying persons with drug addiction are dually diagnosed as having schizophrenia and substance abuse. Biochemically, prolonged drug addiction always results in damage of the central nervous system that can lead to occurrence of symptoms of schizophrenia. A report by related psychiatric outpatients for clients with substance abuse and mental problems in Hong Kong showed that around one-third of the cases who take methylamphetamine (ice) have developed active delusions and hallucinations that could be diagnosed as schizophrenia (Hong Kong government 2002).

The harmful effects of drug addiction leading to the cause of schizophrenia are not only biochemical but also psychosocial. There are some drugs, such as hallucinogens, that once inhaled by the individual induce delusions and hallucinations. Many individuals enjoy such delusive sensory stimulation and become addict to hallucinogens. In some cases, the content of drug-induced hallucinations and delusions may be images or sounds generated from the individuals' unfulfilled wishes, needs, and past experiences that are unconsciously suppressed in normal situations. As these are spontaneously recollected by the individual through heavy addiction of hallucinogens, they can finally become continuous self-generated delusions and hallucinations even without taking hallucinogens. At that moment, individuals are undergoing a process of psychosis. Another typical psychosocial cause of schizophrenia because of drug addiction is the intake of methylamphetamine (ice). Among various psychosocial concepts of schizophrenia, recent studies showed that clients with schizophrenia suffer from a hyperreflexivity. It is an exaggerated self-consciousness in which a subject or agent itself (Sass and Parnas 2003). That means, individuals with schizophrenia embrace the "flight of idea" with too many thoughts on their minds. All these ideas are actually doubts and uncertainties about one's own sense of existence. As amphetamine is a kind of physical stimulant, prolonged intake of it may cause the individual to become accustomed to having the flight of idea in their thinking. Also, the highly excited mental state actually facilitates the individual to having a diffused sense of self and reality. Gradually, the individual's hyperreflexivity mechanism is formulated. As a consequence, they become more vulnerable to the onset of schizophrenia.

Finally, schizophrenia is possibly a result of traumas induced by drug addiction. It is the breaking effects of traumas. Traumas induced by drug addiction can be a drastic physical deterioration, such as failure of bladder function, malfunctioning of the central nervous system, and other problems in organs. Apart from bodily traumas, there are also different types of interpersonal traumas induced by prolonged drug addiction, such as being sexually raped and molested by others in taking drugs, financial difficulties, unemployment, being excluded by significant others, and rejection by healthy peers and family members. After a prolonged chronic drug addiction, some clients may even become homeless street sleepers. All these have a breaking effect of the self-system of clients with drug addiction leading to the onset of schizophrenia.

Clinically speaking, there are some cases showing that continuous substance abuse deters or delays the occurrence of schizophrenia. In those sorts of cases, individuals are being oppressed by related parties in their social environment. According to Laing (1960), people with schizophrenia are usually engulfed, imploded, and depersonalized by their significant others, in particular their parents. They need to fracture their self-system into true and false self. That means, the false and unembodied self is clinically dead by others' engulfment, depersonalization, and implosion so that the true self can be alive within the self-constructed and delusive reality. Within this line of thinking, individuals with drug addiction use the physical and mental stimulation to help the individual temporarily escape from the engulfing, imploding, and depersonalizing reality. That means, the effects of drugs create a temporarily "drug-induced false self" to rescue the individual from the engulfing, imploding, and depersonalizing reality. In doing so, the process of self-fragmentation is delayed by the drug addiction, but the harmful effects of the drug are deepened.

Drug Addiction and Depression

For individuals with prolonged and chronic drug addiction, their mood is easily disturbed and fluctuated by the effects of drug. Most of them may feel highly frustrated, anxious, confused, and empty about difficulties, traumas, and suffering in life. They incline to use drugs as an immediate way to pull up their mood by taking amphetamines, to feel extremely relaxed and released by taking heroine, to feel being free from the painful world by taking ketamines, and to feel delusively excited by taking hallucinogens. However, when the stimulating effects of drugs are over, they have to return to the painful world that can be even more depressive, frustrating, and painful. As a consequence, their emotions become highly fluctuating and confused. In addition to that, as the individual takes drugs for a long while, his/her body may develop tolerance effects on the drug s/he takes. For some drugs such as heroin and cocaine, individual users may also have intolerable withdrawal effects, making the individual crave the drug. Within all these withdrawal effects, individuals consist of both physiological symptoms as well as psychological symptoms. Physiological symptoms make the individual feel a lot of painful and discomfort, so s/he needs to take drugs immediately so as to release all these physiological withdrawal symptoms. Psychological withdrawal symptoms always consist of tensions, restlessness, and severe depressive symptoms. In some types of drugs, such as ketamines and hallucinogens, physiological withdrawal symptoms are absent, but psychological withdrawal still prevail. That means, depressive symptoms are commonly included in psychological withdrawal symptoms in substance abuse.

Similar to the relationship between schizophrenia and drug addiction, depression and drug addiction can go both ways. On one hand, drug addiction leads to a depressive mood. As withdrawal symptoms consist of a depressive mood, the more chronic drug addiction is, the more severe the withdrawal symptoms and the more serious the depressive mood. On the other hand, drug addiction, in particular alcohol, is able to help others in dealing with their depressive moods. When people feel depressed, empty, and frustrated, they are accustomed to heavily drinking alcohol. When they get drunk, their sense of frustration is deeply alleviated. In other words, the drug addiction enables them to get away from their sense of frustration so that they can face the frustrating reality again.

Apart from psychological withdrawal symptoms, severe depression also occurs in traumatic loss caused by chronic drug addiction. As mentioned above, prolonged drug addiction may lead to traumatic loss of employment, property, family members, prestige, status, and identity. All these traumatic losses nurture the depressive mood, in which the individual dreadfully thinks s/he is no longer a complete person after the loss of employment, family members, status, and job.

Drug Addiction and Borderline Personality Disorder

Drug addiction is closely related to BPD. The major symptom of borderline personality disorder is instability in the self-image, affect, and interpersonal relationship. Related theories showed that people with borderline personality suffer from abandonment trauma in their early life. In fact, BPD and drug addiction can be mutually reinforcing to one another. On one hand, people who suffer from BPD may be inclined to use drugs to ease out their sense of frustration and smooth out their emotional fluctuation. On the other hand, the traumatic effects of drug addiction may also increase their vulnerability to abandonment trauma. Because of prolonged chronic drug addiction, they are abandoned by their family members, peers, colleagues, and schoolmates before the onset of their drug addiction. They become more and more lonely and desperate in their life. Gradually, they are more and more adhesive to their drug-related peers. In some cases, in particular female clients with BPD, they are very attached to their drug-addicted boyfriend. To gain and maintain their attachment with her boyfriend, she takes drugs with him. Drug addiction becomes their media for attachment and courtship. In some cases, drug addiction is a replaced substituted attachment in life. The more they are abandoned by their caregivers, the more they need and are inclined to drug addiction as their only substituted attachment object, and the more their fluctuating and unstable their affect, relationship, and self-image become.

Drug Addiction and Neurosis

Drug addiction and neurosis are closely related to one another. Nearly most clients with drug addiction harbor tension, worries, and anxiety in life. As most of them do not harbor sufficient resources, social network, and problem-solving abilities to face these tensions, drug addiction and substance abuse become their own way to face all this. In pathological terms, clients with prolonged drug addiction seem to have a high level of anxiety and worry that are suppressed and repressed by the effects of drug intake. For instance, for those with depressive moods, the effect of stimulants such as amphetamines may help the individual to pull up their depressive mood. For those with intensive anxiety and worries, the taking of ketamines may help them to ease out their anxiety, in particular within their "out-of-body experiences." However, prolonged drug addiction, because of drug-induced traumas, may also increase clients' stress, worries, and anxieties. As a consequence, they may need a higher dosage to suppress all these increased worries and anxiety.

TRAUMA, MENTAL ILLNESS, AND DRUG ADDICTION

As mentioned above, there is a highly complicated relationship among trauma, mental illness, and drug addiction. To have a comprehensive discussion on that, we have the following clarification. First, there are two main types of traumas: non-drug-related trauma (T) and drug-induced trauma (Td). Second, there are two causes of mental illness: non-drug-related mental illness (M) and drug-induced mental illness (Md). All these have a substantial influence or are being influenced by drug addiction (D). With this clarification, the relationship of trauma, mental illness, and drug addiction can be summed up in the following conditions:

1. T leads to M. D is used to cope with M and T.
2. D is used to cope with T. Prolonged D leads to Td and related Md.
3. D is used to cope with M. Prolonged D leads to Td and related Md.
4. D leads to Md and Td, further intensive D to cope with Md and Td.

Regarding the first condition (T leads to M. D is used to cope with M and T), related traumas in life, such as being abandoned, abused, bullied, or humiliated by one's family members, peers, and friends, make the individual suffer from various types of mental problems, such as severe anxiety, tension, stress, or even inclination to major depressive disorder, BPD, or PTSD. However, with all these mental problems being manifested, the individual faces insurmountable stress and difficulties with possible mental and emotional confusion. In facing all these, the individual engages in spontaneous drug addiction to alleviate their stress and mental and emotional confusion and disturbance. Gradually, the individual is accustomed to using drug addiction as the only means to face his or her mental stress and confused mental and emotional state.

For the second condition (D is used to cope with T. Prolonged D leads to Td and related Md), drug addiction is used to cope with trauma and stress in life. These traumas can be physical abuse and abandonment, as well as oppression by significant others in childhood, adolescence, and adulthood. However, because of the harmful effects of drug addiction, individuals suffer a lot from drug-induced traumas, such as being socially isolated by others, financial difficulties, unemployment, and deteriorating body condition and health. In addition to this, prolonged drug addiction also leads to different types of mental problems: (1) schizophrenia because of the physical destructive effect of drugs on the central nervous system, as well as the prolonged social isolation and detachment from reality; (2) depression due to withdrawal effects of drug taking; (3) prolonged anxiety in facing life stress and drug-induced stress and traumas; and (4) PTSD in facing drug-induced traumas.

The third condition (D is used to cope with M. Prolonged D leads to Td and related Md) is that drug addiction is used to cope with mental illness. It delays the onset of various kinds of mental problems. For example, for clients with BPD who suffer from abandonment trauma in their life development, drugs and drug-related peers become kinds of substitute attachment objects to gratify their attachment hunger. In doing so, their emotional fluctuation may be stabilized. Similarly, many clients may regard alcohol addiction as an effective means to paralyze their severe depressive mood generated from frustration in life. However, prolonged drug addiction weakens and deteriorates the client's mental and physical condition to a stage that leads to the onset of mental illness. In this condition, there may be two situations. The first situation is that the mental problems delayed by the drug addiction are similar to the mental problems provoked by prolonged traumas, as well as by deteriorating mental and physical conditions induced by prolonged drug addiction. The second situation is mental problems delayed by the drug addiction are different from the mental problems provoked by prolonged traumas, as well as deteriorating mental and physical conditions induced by prolonged drug addiction. These two situations can be represented in the following conditions:

D is used to cope with M1. Prolonged D leads to Td and related Md (similar to M1)

D is used to cope with M1. Prolonged D leads to Td and related Md (M2, different from M1)

In the fourth condition (D leads to Md and Td, further intensive D to cope with Md and Td), prolonged drug addiction leads to drug-induced mental illness and traumas. However, as the individual does not have any way to cope with related mental illness and trauma, further intensive drug addiction seems to be the only alternative to cope with the mental and physical pain due to drug-induced trauma and physical and mental problems. This is an endless vicious cycle with more and more severe drug-induced traumas and mental problems, that is, unless the client seeks external help in detoxification, harm reduction, or proper treatment of their mental and physical problems. Otherwise, the vicious cycle goes on until one of following endings:

1. The client suffers from a highly confused mental breakdown, mostly schizophrenia, in which he is seriously out of touch of reality.
2. Overdosage of intensive and frequent intake of drug ends up by a final fatal consequence.
3. Committing suicide to end up his/her life so as to end the endless pain and drug addiction.

4. Severe and terminal physical illness in a way that the individual can no longer take drugs because his poor physical condition disables him/her to obtain drugs.

Before the final ending, many clients with drug addiction may fully be aware that this is an endless vicious cycle. At that moment, the client with drug addiction has lost nearly everything (employment, fortune, peers, family members, and dignity) in his/her life. At this rock bottom, some clients are determined to seek help from related professionals. Instead of waiting for their end, they prefer to be admitted to a drug detoxification center, mental hospital, or residential drug rehabilitation center.

Similar to the above-mentioned relationship between drug addiction and trauma, these four conditions appear in different stages of drug addiction. The first condition should manifest before and immediately after initial drug addiction and substance abuse (T leads to M. D is used to cope with M and T). That means, before the client engages in drug addiction and substance abuse, they may suffer from trauma and mental illness. When the individual becomes a regular user, prolonged drug addiction tends to create both mental and physical deterioration on the individual. At that situation, condition 2 and condition 3 occur. In condition 2, drug addiction is used to cope with developmental traumas; however, prolonged drug addiction leads to drug-induced traumas and mental illness. In condition 3, drug addiction is used to cope with mental illness; however, prolonged drug addiction leads to induced traumas and mental illness. Related mental illness induced by prolonged drug addiction can be similar or different from those before drug addiction.

In many ways, condition 2 and condition 3 always happen together. As a regular user of drug, the individual is actually keeping a very delicate and fragile balance between the coping and the destructive effects of drugs. On one hand, it helps the individual to cope with trauma and mental problems. On the other hand, it creates further mental and physical deterioration.

For regular users, those who have used for many years without too much mental or physical deterioration, the individual actually adjusts his/her dosage according to his/her stress level. When s/he is too pressed or frustrated by traumas and/or mental problems induced by drugs or occurring in different life stages, s/he may take a higher dosage to counteract his/her inner pain and frustration. When his/her life stress is lightened, s/he may adjust his/her dosage of the drug to a maintaining level.

However, there are times that the individual is out of control in his/her life. It can be unexpected difficulties and hardship, such as being abandoned by one's spouse, family, unpredictable occurrence of diseases, and death of family members. All these are unbearable for clients with drug addiction. To cope with their unexpected difficulties and hardship, the individual can only use more serious drugs. As a consequence, the individual changes from a regular user to a chronic user. In doing so, his/her drug-induced traumas and mental illness prevail. That means, s/he is in condition 4 (D leads to Md and Td, further intensive D to cope with Md and Td). That is, drug addiction leads to drug-induced mental illness and traumas. Further intensification of drug addiction is needed to cope with all these drug-induced mental illnesses and traumas.

The chronic users, as mentioned above, if they do not have any awareness at rock bottom to seek external help in detoxification, treatment, and recovery, they may finally end up with severe mental illness, severe physical illness, suicide, or sudden death due to an overdose of drugs. All these can be summarized in the following table 2.

Table 2: Conditions of Trauma and Mental Illness in Different Degress of Drug Addiciton

Types of Users	Conditions of Trauma, Mental Illness, and Drug Addiction
Initial Users	T leads to M. D is used to cope with M and T (Condition 1).
Regular Users	D is used to cope with T. Prolonged D leads to Td and related Md (Condition 2), and D is used to cope with M. Prolonged D leads to Td and related Md (Condition 3).
Chronic Users	D leads to Md and Td, further intensive D to cope with Md and Td (Condition 4).

CONCLUSION

This chapter has outlined the initial theoretical frame on trauma, mental illness, and drug addiction. The writer outlines two forces in people with drug addiction. Force A is that drug addiction provides a temporary coping and escape for individuals to face traumas, sufferings and hardships in life, and delay the onset of possible mental problems. Force B is prolonged drug addiction that provokes and induces related traumas leading to physical and mental deterioration, including severe mental problems. These two forces interact with one another in various ways in different stages of drug addiction.

Stage 1: Force A Only (Initial or Occasional Users)

Stage 2: Force A Inhibits Force B (Regular Users: Initial Addiction)

Stage 3: Force A Combines with Force B (Long-Term Regular Users: Full Addiction)

Stage 4: Force A Reinforces Force B (Chronic Addiction)

Stage 5: Force B Inhibits Force A (Rock Bottom of Chronic Addiction)

Apart from Force A and Force B, there are also other forces in governing the drug addiction and substance abuse. Force C and Force D concerns with the sense of subjectivity in the process of drug addiction. Force C is the drug-induced sense of subjectivity. Force D is the sense of subjectivity being deteriorated in prolonged drug addiction. Forces C and D intermingle with one another in the process of drug addiction as Force A and B. Force E is the drug-induced sense of reality.

Force F is the sense of reality being gradually eroded by prolonged drug addiction. Similarly, Force E and F interact with one another as Force A and B. In other words, these three pairs of forces, A and B, C and D, and E and F all interact with one another, shaping the individual's trauma and resilience, sense of subjectivity, and sense of reality in the process of drug addiction.

Furthermore, the writer describes a comprehensive process of traumatization with the following elements and components:

- Natures of Trauma: people involved (A), related events (B), duration (C)
- Immediate Effects of Trauma: acute stress disorder (D)
- Prolonged Effect: Rebound and Recall of Traumatic Experiences: Post-traumatic Stress Disorder (Recollection) (E)
- Prolonged Effect: Avoidance and further suppression of Recall of Traumatic Experiences: Post-Traumatic Stress Disorder (Avoidance) (F)
- Prolonged Effect: Increase of Arousal in Traumatic Disturbance: Post-Traumatic Stress Disorder (Increase in arousal) (G)
- Chronic Effect of Trauma: Breaking Effect (H)
- Chronic Effect of Trauma: Loss Effect (I)
- Chronic Effects of Trauma: Awakening of Unpleasant Repression (J)
- Chronic Effects of Trauma: Wounded Self (K)

From the above-mentioned discussion, it is clear that acute effects, rebound, and recall effects, as well as the chronic effects of trauma, all have a close relationship with the onset of various types of mental illness.

Acute Effect = Acute Stress Disorder and Dissociative Disorder

Recall, Avoidance, and Arousal of Disturbance = Post-Traumatic Stress Disorder

Chronic Effects: the Loss Effect = Depression and Major Depressive Disorder

Chronic Effects: the Breaking Effect = Schizophrenia and Dissociative Disorder

Chronic Effects: the Awakening Effect = Anxiety Disorders

Chronic Effects: the Wounded Self = Personality Disorder

Prolonged drug addiction has a high co-morbidity with different types of mental illness. Conceptually, there may be three different types of positions regarding the relationship between mental illness and drug addiction. They are listed as follows:

1. Prolonged drug addiction leads to various types of mental illnesses.
2. Mental illness or problems are coped with and delayed by spontaneous drug addiction.
3. Drug addiction goes together with various types of mental illnesses or problems.

Regarding position 1, drug addiction leads to various types of mental illnesses; there can be three different types of causes:

1A. Prolonged drug addiction creates irreversible harm to the central nervous system and leads to mental confusion and occurrence of different types of mental illnesses, in particular schizophrenia.

1B. Prolonged drug addiction nurtures drug-related interpersonal and psychosocial traumas that lead to occurrence of different types of mental illnesses, in particular depression, BPD, and schizophrenia.

1C. Prolonged drug addiction creates irreversible harm to organs such as the liver, bladder, and kidneys. Deterioration and failure of organs nurture mental stress to the individual with a result of mental problems.

Regarding position 2, mental illnesses or mental problems are delayed or can be coped with by drug addiction. It can be done in several ways.

2A. Drug addiction enables the individual to escape from the painfully oppressive reality; thus, delayed mental illnesses nurtures by oppressive reality.

2B. Drug addiction provides the individual a means to suppress and repress the recall and rebound of various kinds of traumas that provoke various types of mental illnesses or mental problems.

2C. Drug addiction alters the state of mind and body of the individual. At the same time, it also alters the individual's psychosocial and physical condition that leads to certain types of mental illnesses or mental problems.

Regarding position 3, drug addiction goes together with various types of mental illnesses or mental problems, it can also happen in several ways.

3A. Mental illnesses or problems occur before the intake of drugs (mixing with the withdrawal effects of drugs).

3B. Mental illnesses or problems occur during the intake of drugs (co-morbid with the stimulating effects of drugs).

3C. Mental illnesses or problems occur immediate after the intake of drugs (co-morbid with after the diminishing of the stimulating effects of drugs).

3D. Mental illness or problems occur long after the intake of drugs.

Chapter 3

Understanding and Intervention for People with Drug Addiction, Abandonment Trauma, and Borderline Personality Disorder

Introduction

Abandonment trauma commonly occurs in people with chronic drug addiction. Many of them have a painful childhood and adolescence in which they are neglected, separated, abused, and oppressed by their significant others. For them, drug addiction and substance abuse merely serve three purposes and functions. First, it is used a substituted attachment object. In real life, they fail to attach to anyone. Everyone leaves and separates from them. In prolonged and chronic drug addiction, individuals use drugs as a substituted attachment object. Second, it serves as a means to relate to other drug-related peers or significant others. That means, by taking drugs, they can relate to their peers, siblings, boyfriends/girlfriends, or even their parents with drug addiction. In other words, they are dreadfully lonely and empty in life. Apart from being abandoned by their significant others in childhood and adolescence, they may also be rejected and excluded from their friends, colleagues, family members, or spouses. They have no one to turn to and interact with in daily life.

Below is the self-narration of client A with a chronic drug addiction demonstrating the dreadful sense of loneliness and dependence on drug addiction as the only reliance in life.

> A: I have been taking "ice" and "ketamine" for over ten years. At first, I thought taking ice gave me some strange and wonderful experience. I tried this and found it was very exciting. In particular, it helped to alleviate my depressive and lonely mood. I came from a single-parent family in which my mother died when I was only two years old. My father took care of me, but he was busy traveling around mainland China and Hong Kong. He never had time to be with me in childhood and adolescence. I lived with my aunt and uncle. But they did not care for me much. They took care of me simply because my father could give them a significant amount of money so that they could have enough income to nurture their four children. As I was not cared for by my parents, they looked down upon me. My nephews even bullied me in front of others. I was dreadfully lonely and sad. I wanted to attack to my teachers and my classmates in school. But most of them were realistic and calculating. They simply wanted my father to give them some reward or benefit before they really cared about me. So, I only approached peers who were also uncared for or even rejected by their families. Gradually, I had nowhere to go except to take ice and adhere to my drug-related peers. We took drugs together. We enjoyed being "confused" or "stimulated" by drugs. When we had taken ice, we felt so high and did anything. Sometimes, sex went with drug addiction. At first, my father and my aunt did not know that. Later, my classmate told my teacher that I was a drug user. She disclosed that to my aunt and my father. They were furious. I argued with them. I left my aunt's house and accompanied my boyfriend who was a delinquent. We took ice together. Sex and drugs became our daily activities. He finally left me and found another girl. I hated him. I found another boyfriend and shifted to ketamines, simply because he liked it.
>
> Two years later, he got along with another girl and abandoned me. At that moment, I had already become a regular drug user. Apart from taking drugs, I did not have any companionship. That means, the drug was my only companion.

> In all those years, I was lonely and depressed. In fact, no one could really understand us, including teachers, social workers, psychiatrists, and psychologists. They only thought I was a subject for diagnosis, assessment, and so-called intervention. Some of them introduced the toxic effects of drugs to me. In fact, I knew that much more than they did.

From A's self-narration, it was clear that A was dreadfully lonely and suffered a lot from her abandonment traumas in life. The first abandonment trauma started with the death of her mother and prolonged emotional neglect of her father. Second, she was spontaneously bullied and ignored both by her nephews, uncle, and aunt. She had no one to turn to when she felt lonely, oppressed, and frustrated in life. In other words, drugs and drug-related peers were the only means and media for her to turn to. According to a DSM IV diagnosis, client A suffered from BPD in which abandonment traumas in childhood and adolescence made A have instability in affect, cognition, relationship, and self-image. In this chapter, the writer discusses related interpretation and intervention for people with drug addiction, abandonment trauma, and BPD.

Diagnosis and Etiology of Borderline Personality Disorder

BPD is a common and severe personality disorder with the following diagnosis from both DSM IV and DSM V:

Diagnostic Criteria

> A pervasive pattern of instability of interpersonal relationship, self-image, and affects, and marked impulsivity beginning by early adulthood and present in a variety of contexts, as indicated by five (or more) of the following:

1) Frantic efforts to avoid real or imagined abandonment. Note: Do not include suicidal or self-mutilation behavior covered in Criterion 5
2) A pattern of unstable and intense interpersonal relationships characterized by alternating between extremes of idealization and devaluation
3) Identity disturbance: markedly and persistently unstable self-image or sense of self
4) Impulsivity in at least two areas that are potentially self-damaging (e.g., spending, sex, substance abuse, reckless driving, binge eating) Note: Do not include suicidal or self-mutilating behavior
5) Recurrent suicidal behavior, gestures, threats, or self-mutilating behavior
6) Affective instability due to a marked reactivity of mood
7) Chronic feeling of emptiness
8) Inappropriate, intense anger or difficulty controlling anger
9) Transient, stress-related paranoid ideation or severe dissociative symptoms

(American Psychiatric Association 1994: 650–4)

Etiology

A careful articulation of these nine symptoms can be grouped into three groups:

As mentioned above, there are three sorts of symptoms in BPD. They are:

1) Problems in Personality Structures (symptoms 1, 2, 3)

Frantic efforts to avoid real or imagined abandonment. Note: Do not include suicidal or self-mutilation behaviour covered in Criterion 5 (Symptom 1)

A pattern of unstable and intense interpersonal relationships characterized by alternating between extremes of idealization and devaluation (Symptom 2)

Identity disturbance; markedly and persistently unstable self-image or sense of self (Symptom 3)

2) Impulsive Mood, Uncontrollable Anger and Self-Harm Behaviors (Symptoms 4, 5, 6 & 8)

Impulsivity in at least two areas that are potentially self-damaging (e.g., spending, sex, substance abuse, reckless driving, binge eating) Note: Do not include suicidal or self-mutilating behavior (Symptom 4)

Recurrent suicidal behavior, gestures, or threats, or self-mutilating behavior (Symptom 5)

Affective instability due to a marked reactivity of mood (Symptom 6)

Inappropriate, intense anger or difficulty controlling anger (Symptom 8)

3) Chronic Emptiness, Paranoid Ideation and Dissociative Symptoms (Symptoms 7 & 9)

Chronic feeling of emptiness (Symptom 7)

Transient, stress-related paranoid ideation (Symptom 9a)

Severe dissociative symptoms (Symptom 9b)

Personality Structure Problems Due to Primary Abandonment Traumas

The first group of symptoms (1, 2, and 3) implies that the individual suffers a lot of related abandonment traumas in their infancy, childhood, and adolescence in which they fail to establish a regular, constant, and trustworthy relationship with others. They become highly insecure and anxious in relating to others. Any mild or temporary separation, loss, rejection, or criticism may trigger their former abandonment trauma, making them become highly fluctuating and impulsive in perceiving oneself and others. Very often, this sort of instability in interpersonal relationship and self-image can last for their whole life.

Traumas, Emotional Neglect, and Abandonment in Childhood and Adolescence

Related studies show that people with BPD encounter traumas in their childhood or adolescence such as abandonment, sex trauma, domestic violence, and abuse (McGlashan 1985; Herman et al. 1989; Links and

Steiner 1988). Some even have adoption, early parental loss, and incest trauma (McGlashan 1985). The most severe borderline patients suffered from sexual abuse, usually when very young (Links and Steiner 1988). The Herman et al. (1989) study demonstrated that subjects with BPD suffered from childhood trauma (81%), physical abuse (71%), sex abuse (68%), or witnessed serious domestic violence (62%). Herman et al. (1989) argued that BPD is similar to PTSD.

Briere (1992) cited National Center of Child Abuse and Neglect (1990) studied 200,000 cases of child abuse and discovered that there were eight types of psychological abuse imposed by caretakers.

> 1) Rejecting: The child is avoided or pushed away, s/he is made to feel unworthy, unacceptable and the like.
> 2) Degrading/devaluating: The child is criticized, stigmatized, deprived of dignity, humiliated, made to feel inferior and so on.
> 3) Terrorizing: The child is verbally assaulted, frightened, threatened with physical or psychological harm.
> 4) Isolating: The child is deprived of social contacts beyond the family, not allow friends, kept in limited areas for long periods of time without social interaction.
> 5) Corrupting: The child is socialized and taught to behave in an antisocial manner, encouraged to develop socially unacceptable interests and appetites.
> 6) Exploiting: The child is taken advantage of, used to meet the needs of his/her caretaker.
> 7) Denying essential stimulation, emotional responsiveness or availability: The child is deprived of loving, sensitive caregiving: his/her emotional and intellectual development is stifled, the child is generally ignored or neglected.
> 8) Unreliable and inconsistent parenting: Contradictory and ambivalent demand are made of the child, parental support or caregiving is inconsistent and unreliable, and familial stability is denied the child.
>
> (Briere 1992: 9–10)

In other words, within these eight types of psychological abuse, children may think that they are merely subjects for exploitation and abuse. Even though their parents or caretakers live with them, they do not feel any love and concern. In terms of love and affection, they are emotionally abandoned by their parents and caretakers (Yip 2013).

Emotional neglect is defined as:

> Act of omission, frequently the result of parental ignorance or indifference. As a result, the child is not given positive emotional support and stimulation. Parents may give adequate physical care to their child but leave him/her alone in a crib for long period of time, seldom cuddle or talk to the child, or fail to give him/her encouragement and recognition. (Briere 1992: 15)

Within all this psychological abuse and emotional neglect, children actually live within a prolonged and highly traumatic social environment with a highly destructive impact on their development of selfhood and personality structure. On one hand, they hate their significant others who abandon or psychological abuse them. On the other hand, they need to attach to their significant others as much as possible to fulfill their developmental needs. Furthermore, they may presume that either they are so bad that their significant others abandon them or they are good but their significant others are bad and abandon them. If their significant others leave them permanently, they conclude that their significant others are bad and abandon them. However, if their caretakers emotionally neglect and psychologically abuse them but still attach to them, this conflicting presumption persists in their developmental process. Together with this is also the prevailing fear of being abandoned by others and anger toward real or imagined abandonment as described in the diagnosis criteria.

> The perception of impending separation or rejection, or the loss of external structure can lead to profound changes in self-image, affect, cognition, and behavior. These individuals are very sensitive to environmental circumstances. They experience intense abandonment fears and inappropriate anger even when faced with a realistic time limited

> separation or when there are unavoidable changes in plans. They believe that this abandonment implies they are "bad." Their frantic effort to avoid abandonment may include impulsive actions such as self-mutilating or suicidal behaviors. (American Psychiatric Association 1994: 650)

From the above-mentioned diagnosis of BPD, it is clear that the abandonment trauma that happened in the individual's childhood has a profound negative effect on his/her development. The loss of external structure implies that the individual is unable to develop stable personality organization with a result of unstable self-image, affect, cognition, and relationship. They become highly sensitive to interpersonal relationships. As they have suffered from abandonment trauma, they harbor irrational fear toward separation. They cannot tolerate even temporary separation within a short time limit and avoid changes in plans. They simply regard any separation implies abandonment. They project their anger of childhood abandonment toward anyone whom they regard is going to, or appears to, separate from them (Yip 2013).

In other words, in facing this sort of abandonment trauma in childhood, individuals with BPD become highly sensitive to real or imagined abandonment. Even in temporary separation with their significant others, they may have the following responses:

1) They may come to a conclusion they are bad that others abandon them.
2) They may assume that others (their parents) are bad that they abandon them.
3) They may fluctuate from these two assumptions (whether they are bad or others are bad in abandonment).
4) Within this fluctuation, individuals feel angry towards themselves and significant others. They also harbor intensive fear towards actual and imagined abandonment.
5) Within intensive anger and fear, individuals are highly sensitive and fluctuating to interpersonal relationships. (Yip 2013)

Attachment Hunger, Abandonment Fear and Anger

Abandonment trauma, because of emotional neglect from caregivers or parents, creates three inter-related problems in clients' lives. They are:

1) *Attachment hunger:* Clients earnestly urge for attachment to substituted attachment figures so as to fulfill their ungratified need of attachment in early life.
2) *Abandonment fear:* In relating to others, they harbor intensive fear that sooner or later, they will be abandoned by them.
3) *Abandonment anger:* In relating to others, their hidden anger of being abandoned by caregivers is easily triggered. (Yip 2013)

These three problems intermingle with one another formulating unresolved emotional dilemmas that may finally lead to fluctuating emotions and relationships. They are:

A: Approach and Avoidance Dilemma:

When attachment hunger intermingles with abandonment fear, individuals urge to connect with substituted attachment figures on one hand, but harbor an intensive fear that sooner or later they would be abandoned. That means, they want to get close to others, but they dare not to get too close to avoid being abandoned. (Yip, 2013)

B: Love and Hate Dilemma:

When attachment hunger intermingles with abandonment anger, individuals urge to connect with substituted attachment figures on one hand. When they get too close to others, their abandonment anger in early life is triggered. Thus, they easily project this unresolved anger towards the substituted attachment figure. That means, they love to connect with others but easily become angry in facing others' mild comment, criticism, and separation. (Yip 2013).

C: Explosive Anger and Repressed Fear Confusion:

Abandonment fear and abandonment anger inhibits one another. When individuals' abandonment anger is triggered, they may throw their anger towards their substituted attachment figures. However, their fear of abandonment may inhibit them to do so. However, the anger does not vanish. Instead, it accumulates until an intolerable level. At the moment, individuals may suddenly blow up their anger explosively towards others. However, after the temperament, their abandonment fear makes them feel deep regret, thinking that the explosion of anger may finally lead to the leaving of substituted attachment figures. (Yip, 2013)

Instability in Perception of Self and Others

Instability in Perception of Others

According to the diagnosis of BPD given in DSM IV, persons with BPD can have an intensive fluctuation of both self-image and the perception of others.

> They may idealize potential caregivers or lovers at the first or second meeting, demand to spend a lot of time together, and share most intimate details early in a relationship. However, they may switch quickly from idealizing other people to devaluing them, feeling that the other person does not care enough, does not give enough, is not "there" enough. These individuals can empathize with and nurture other people, but only with the expectation that the other person will "be there" in return to meet their own needs on demand. These individuals are prone to sudden and dramatic shifts in their view of others, who may alternately be seen as beneficent supports or as cruelly punitive. Such shifts often reflect disillusionment with a caregiver whose nurturing qualities had been idealized or whose rejection or abandonment is expected. (American Psychiatric Association 1994: 650)

Within the DSM IV diagnosis, it is clear that persons with BPD tend to have a contrasting view on others. At one time, they perceive others with idealizing and caring to whom they attach to and build up intimate relationship with. At another time, they tend to devaluate others, feeling that others are not caring and even trying to reject and separate from them. The shifting of idealizing and devaluating toward others can occur suddenly according to their own demands and needs. The shifting of devaluation and idealizing is particularly imposed on related caregivers' caring qualities. In the idealizing situation, persons with BPD are highly attached to their caregivers and appreciate their nurturing qualities. In the devaluating situation, they condemn or criticize their caregivers, fearing that sooner or later their caregivers will abandon them. They become highly sensitive to possible or even imagined abandonment in terms of temporary separation, slight rejection, or mild comment by others (Yip 2013).

Instability in Self-Perception

Apart from devaluation and idealizing others, in particular caregivers, persons with BPD also have a dramatic shift in self-images.

> There are sudden and dramatic shifts in self-image, characterized by shifting goals, values, and vocational aspirations. There may be sudden changes in opinions and plans about career, sexual identity, values and types of friends. These individuals may suddenly changes from the role of a needy supplicant for help to a righteous avenger of past maltreatment. Although they usually have a self-image that is based on being bad or evil, individuals with this disorder may at times have feelings that do not exist at all. Such experiences usually occur in situations in which the individual feels a lack of a meaningful relationship, nurturing, and support. These individuals may show worse performance in unstructured work or school situations. (American Psychiatric Association 1994: 651)

According to DSM IV, persons with BPD have a dramatic shift in self-image with the following changes:

1) Shifting of personal goals, opinion, plans of career and vocational aspiration
2) Changes in sexual identity and values

3) Changes from a needy supplicant for help to a righteous avenger of past maltreatment
4) Changes of self-image of being bad or evil
5) Changes of feeling from intensively moody to having no feeling at all

Instability in Perception of Self and Others

According to Yip (2013), it is clear that persons with BPD, under the profound influence of abandonment trauma in childhood, are unable to establish a stable external structure of self-image, identity, morality, and emotionality. Putting the instability in perceiving oneself and others together, persons with BPD should be shifting among the following perception of self and others:

1) Idealization of Self (Si)
2) Devaluation of Self (Sd)
3) Idealization of Other (Oi)
4) Devaluation of Other (Od)

Four Stages in Shifting of Perception of Self and Others

Yip (2013) asserted that there should be four stages in the shifting of perception of self and others for persons with BPD.

Stage 1: Si + Oi (Idealizing intimacy in satisfying attachment hunger for potential caregivers)

Stage 2: Si + Od (Oversensitive and being angry at assumed caregivers' mild comment, criticism, isolation, and separation: imagined abandonment)

Stage 3: Sd + Oi (Devaluating oneself so as to retain the caregivers' possible isolation, separation, or even possible abandonment)

Stage 4: Sd + Od (Complete but intolerable emptiness after the actual separation or leaving by assumed caregivers)

Within these four stages of changes, attachment hunger, abandonment fears, and abandonment anger change accordingly as shown in the following Table 3 by Yip (2013).

Table 3. Attachment Hunger, Abandonment Fear, and Anger in Various Stages by Yip (2013)

Stages	Anxious Attachment and Attachment Hunger	Manifestation of Abandonment Fear	Manifestation of Abandonment Anger
Before the onset of BPD The impact of abandonment traumas: Prolonged failure to develop stable attachment and transitional object	Anxious attachment nurtures attachment hunger to attachment figures	Intensive fear that the attachment figure would be going to leave him/her in infancy, childhood and/or adolescence	Intensive anger that the attachment figure had abandoned him/her in infancy, childhood and/or adolescence
Stage 1: Si + Oi Idealized Self and Idealized Other	Attachment Hunger prevails pushing the individual to cling on substituted attachment figures	Abandonment fear is properly concealed within the prevailing attachment hunger	Abandonment anger is also properly concealed within the prevailing attachment hunger
From Stage 1 to Stage 2 Idealized Other tends to have lot of deficits	Individuals have already attached to substituted figure	Concealed abandonment fear is triggered by some mild comment or temporary separation from the substituted attachment figure	Use abandonment anger to suppress abandonment fear. The anger being rejected by former attachment figure begins to accumulate.
Stage 2: Si + Od Idealized Self and Devaluated Other	Attachment hunger pushes the individual to be intensively dependent on the substituted attachment figure. That may be intolerable for the substituted attachment figure	Fear of being abandoned could not be properly expressed. S/he tries to avoid thinking about that.	Abandonment anger prevails in response to the mild comment, temporary separation and slight rejection from the substituted attachment figure. The individual projects his anger in abandonment traumas towards the substituted attachment figure.

Table 3 (Continued)

Stages	Anxious Attachment and Attachment Hunger	Manifestation of Abandonment Fear	Manifestation of Abandonment Anger
From Stage 2 to Stage 3 Idealized Self is gradually transformed into Devaluated Self	The substituted attachment figure feels intolerable and intends to exclude, criticize, and separate from the individual with BPD	Fear of abandonment is greatly intensified. The previous experiences of being abandoned is gradually triggered.	Once the abandonment anger is fully released. The individual feels guilty and regretted. S/he is afraid that it speeds up the separation and abandonment of the substituted attachment figures
Stage 3: Sd + Oi Devaluated Self and Idealized Other	The attachment hunger enables the individual to humiliate himself or herself so as to retain the substituted attachment figure	Fear of abandonment is fully triggered. The individual even tries all means to humiliate himself/herself including emotional blackmailing by self-harm and even suicidal gestures so to suppress the fear of abandonment	The anger towards others in abandoning him/her begins to turn inwards, the individual feels shameful that the substitute figure abandons him/her. Self-directed anger provokes self-harm or even suicidal gestures
From Stage 3 to Stage 4 Both the Self and Other are not idealized. In reality, they are no good. Good thing and event do not belong to me.	The attachment hunger prevails as the substituted attachment figure leaves the individual	Traumatic fear of abandonment prevails in forms of acute stress disorder in facing the leaving of the substituted attachment figure Severe dissociation of mind and body as well as psychosomatic symptoms occurs.	The abandonment anger not only turns inwards but is also internalized and somatised in the dissociation and psychosomatic symptoms
Stage 4: Sd + Od Devaluated Self and Devaluated Other	The attachment hunger prevails as the substituted attachment figure leaves the individual. As there are no available substituted figures around, the individual certainly	Traumatic fear of abandonment highly intensifies and has breaking effects on the ego system. The individual feels that not only substituted attachment figures reject	Self-directed abandonment anger not only turns inwards and becomes somatic symptoms but also begins to fracture the ego system. It creates intensive breaking

	feels dreadfully empty and meaningless	and leave him/her, other people around are also rejecting and leaving him/her. It can gradually transform into paranoid ideation or even paranoid schizophrenia	effects in which the individual may suffer from temporary self-fragmentation in forms of paranoid delusions and hallucinations
From Stage 4 to Stage 1 The Devaluated Self and Devaluated Other need to change to Idealized Self and Idealized Other in a new environment There are chances and opportunities to find new idealized others in new environment	Intensive senses of emptiness and meaninglessness are intolerable for the individual. As his/her ego is strengthened and system still functional and integrated. The attachment hunger tends to overcome meaninglessness and emptiness The individual changes his job, social circle, or even his self-identity and gender identity to search for possibility of new substituted attachment figures	The prevailing abandonment fear is enlightened as the individual changes to another social environment in which there are new friends, new colleagues, or new peers The individual begins to harbor hope that among these newly encountered persons, there is still someone who is suitable to be his/her potential substituted attachment figure The more s/he focuses on new encountered persons, the more the abandonment fear is enlightened	The heartbreaking abandonment anger is gradually enlightened as the individual changes to a new social environment S/he still harbors a strong hope that people in this new social environment are accepting, caring and supportive As the attachment hunger still prevails, this hope to connect with new potential substituted attachment figures certainly conceals the abandonment anger in this new social environment

Unstable Affect, Impulsive Self-Damaging Behaviors, Anger, and Suicide

The second group of symptoms in BPD consists of unstable affect, uncontrollable anger, suicide, self-mutilation, and self-damaging behaviors.

Affective Instability

Affective instability manifests in forms of the following:

> Affective instability due to a marked reactivity of mood (e.g., intense episode dysphoria, irritability, or anxiety usually lasting a few hours and only rarely more than a few days). The basic dysphoric mood of these individuals is often disrupted by periods of anger, panic, or despair and is rarely relieved by periods of well-being or satisfaction. These episodes may reflect the individual's extreme reactivity to interpersonal stresses. (American Psychiatric Association 1994: 653)

It includes:

1) Intense episode of dysphoria
2) Intense episode of irritability
3) Intense episode of anxiety
4) Intense episode of anger
5) Intense episode of panic

The problem of affective instability exists in several ways:

a) Every episode can be an intense outburst.
b) Every episode can be sudden and unpredictable by others.
c) Every episode lasts for several hours and shifts to another episode (Yip 2013).

Impulsivity

> Impulsivity in at least two areas that are potentially self-damaging (e.g., spending, sex, substance abuse, reckless driving, binge eating). Note: Do not include suicidal or self-mutilating behavior.

Impulsivity occurs in forms of great spending, sex, substance abuse, and recklessness driving. Individuals use such self-damaging behaviors and addiction to release unbearable frustration and anger toward self and others. They are painful coping mechanisms of the real or imagined abandonment from substituted attachment figures. They are ways to detach and disengage from the painful reality; to release or paralyze one's intensive fear and anger in current and past abandonment traumas; and to punish the devaluated self or/and the devaluated others (Yip 2013).

Recurrent Suicidal and Self-Harm Behaviors

> Recurrent suicidal behaviour, gestures, or threats, or self-mutilating behaviour.
>
> Completed suicide occurs in 8%–10% of such individuals, and self-mutilative acts (e.g., cutting or burning) and suicide threats and attempts are common. Recurrent suicidality is often the reason that these individuals present for help. These self-destructive acts are usually precipitated by threats of separation or rejection or by expectations that they assume increased responsibility. Self-mutilation may occur during dissociative experiences and often brings relief by reaffirming the ability to feel or by expiating the individual's sense of being evil. (American Psychiatric Association, 1994: 654)

Strictly speaking, addictive and impulsive behavior, such as substance abuse, great spending, and eating disorders, are also self-harm behaviors. They are used as means for the individual to punish the devaluated self and/or devaluated others. Apart from that, as mentioned above, recurrent suicide and self-destructive acts are precipitated by threats of separation or rejection by others (Yip 2013).

In Stage 3 (Sd + Oi), when the substituted attachment figures are prepared or determined to leave or separate the individual, s/he properly feels desperate and helpless. S/he tries to devaluate himself/herself so as to ask the forgiveness of the substituted attachment figures. S/he may pledge or beg for them to stay. However, if all these cannot be attained. S/he properly feels highly self-humiliated and intolerable as well as angry with the substituted attachment figures. Thus, recurrent suicidality is used as a means for the following purposes:

1) emotional blackmailing of the substituted attachment figures (I will die if you abandon me),

2) taking revenge on the abandonment of the substituted attachment figures (you will finally feel regret for my suicide just because you abandoned me),
3) self-punishment as an ultimate means for self-devaluation (I am nothing, I am always abandoned by others, and I deserve to die), and
4) demonstrating how merciful s/he is so to retain the leave substituted attachment figures (No one cares about me. Even if I die, still no one cares about me. You are caring. Don't you.). (Yip 2013)

In the same way, self-harm behavior, such as covert self-cutting and other self-mutative acts, are performed by the individual for emotional blackmail, to take revenge, to impose self-punishment, and to demonstrate mercy for the substituted attachment figures. For self-cutting, one more functioning is performed; it revitalizes individual's sense of reality. In many cases, the individual feels highly depersonalized before self-harm behaviors. In the process of self-cutting, the individual with BPD feels highly depersonalized and blunt in his/her affect. S/he feels released when s/he sees the blood dripping from his/her wrist (Yip 2013).

Uncontrollable Anger

> Inappropriate, intense anger or difficulty controlling anger (e.g., frequent display of temper, constant anger, recurrent physical fights) (They may display extreme sarcasm, enduring bitterness, or verbal outbursts. The anger is often elicited when a caregiver or lover is seen as neglectful, withholding, uncaring, or abandoning. Such expressions of anger are often followed by shame and guilt and contribute to the feeling they have of being evil). (American Psychiatric Association: 1994: 651–4)

In fact, uncontrollable anger in people with BPD originated from abandonment anger. According to Yip (2013), it can manifest in the following ways:

1) It originates from the abandonment traumas in childhood and adolescence. The individual harbors intense and unexplainable anger as to why his/her attachment figures leaves him/her.

2) The abandonment anger intermingles with abandonment fear toward his/her attachment figures. On one hand, s/he tries to expose his/her anger directly toward his/her attachment figures. On the other hand, s/he is afraid that once this anger is exposed, his/her attachment figures may finally leave him/her. Thus, s/he tends to suppress this abandonment anger by fear.
3) However, the more and the longer the abandonment anger is suppressed by fear, the easier the anger is being triggered and provoked.
4) The abandonment traumas in childhood and adolescence lead to attachment hunger to substituted attachment figures in later life stages. All this deep-seated anger and fear in abandonment trauma are easily projected into the substituted attachment figures in later life stages. In some cases, they also extend to relationships in aging.
5) Anger and fear of abandonment traumas in childhood are easily triggered in various stages of development in BPD.

Chronic Emptiness, Paranoid Ideation, and Dissociative Symptoms

According to DSM IV, chronic emptiness, paranoid ideation, and dissociative symptoms are also important symptoms for people with BPD. They are listed as follows:

> Chronic feeling of emptiness (easily bored, they may constantly seek something to do, these things may be in forms of bad and unhealthy habits).
>
> Transient, stress-related paranoid ideation or severe dissociative symptoms.
>
> (During period of extreme stress, transient paranoid ideation or dissociative symptoms, e.g., depersonalization may occur, but these are generally of sufficient severity or duration to warrant an additional diagnosis. These episodes occur most frequently in response to a real or imagined abandonment. Symptoms tend to be transient, lasting minutes or hours. The real or perceived return of the caregivers' nurturance may result in a remission of symptoms).
>
> (American Psychiatric Association 1994: 650–4)

People with BPD are abandoned in numerous primary abandonment traumas in childhood and infancy, self-induced abandonment in explosive abandonment anger, and fear toward their substituted attachment figures in later life. All these abandonment traumas not only rid them of their psychic and mental energy but also make clients feel dreadfully empty and sense meaningless in life. The dreadful sense of emptiness is particular explicit at the time when their substituted attachment figure leaves them. They earnestly to search for another substituted attachment figure, but they find no one.

The fear of being permanently lonely and empty is also internalized into the body and turns into somatic complaints as well as dissociative symptoms, such hysteria, amnesia, and eating disorders. Coupling this is also an extension of self-hate and self-isolation, as well as paranoid ideation saying that they are not lovable and not respected by others. In some cases, in people with BPD, paranoid ideation can turn into paranoid delusion that can be diagnosed as paranoid schizophrenia.

Different Types of Borderline Conditions

Clinically, people with borderline personality features and inclination can be grouped into four types of borderline conditions: They are:

1) Pre-Borderline Condition
2) Full Energy Borderline Condition
3) Low Energy Borderline Condition
4) Post-Borderline Condition

In different types of borderline conditions, various groups of symptoms are manifested.

Once again, we first review different symptoms of BPD.

> A pervasive pattern of instability of interpersonal relationship, self-image, and affects, and marked impulsivity beginning by early adulthood and present in a variety of contexts, as indicated by five (or more) of the following:

1) Frantic efforts to avoid real or imagined abandonment. Note: Do not include suicidal or self-mutilation behavior covered in Criterion 5
2) A pattern of unstable and intense interpersonal relationships characterized by alternating between extremes of idealization and devaluation
3) Identity disturbance: markedly and persistently unstable self-image or sense of self
4) Impulsivity in at least two areas that are potentially self-damaging (e.g., spending, sex, substance abuse, reckless driving, binge eating) Note: Do not include suicidal or self-mutilating behavior.
5) Recurrent suicidal behavior, gestures, or threats, or self-mutilating behavior.
6) Affective instability due to a marked reactivity of mood
7) Chronic feeling of emptiness
8) Inappropriate, intense anger or difficulty controlling anger
9) Transient, stress-related paranoid ideation or severe dissociative symptoms

(American Psychiatric Association 1994: 650–4)

In pre-borderline condition, clients suffer from primary abandonment traumas in their early life. Clinically, only symptoms 1, 2, and 3 are manifested. Yip (2013) articulated that they symptoms 1, 2, and 3 are problems in personality structure caused by abandonment traumas in which the individual harbors a strong attachment hunger toward substituted attachment figures.

They are unstable in their self-identity as well as in interpersonal relationships. Occasionally, they may have uncontrollable anger or unstable affect, but they are not sufficient to have five symptoms that can be classified as BPD.

In full-energy borderline condition, apart from personality structure problems (symptoms 1, 2, and 3), the client usually manifests outburst of intense anger (symptom 8) (abandonment anger), instable affect (symptom 6), self-damaging behaviors (symptom 4), and even suicidal gestures (symptom 5).

Apart from primary abandonment trauma (TA1), individuals also suffer from secondary or self-induced abandonment trauma (TA2) in which their outburst of anger, instable affect, suicidal gestures, and self-damaging behaviors threaten and provoke the separation and leaving of their substituted attachment figures. It also causes a lot of trouble and resistance in professional intervention.

Many professionals, in particular those inclined to crisis intervention and social control, may regard all these as psychiatric emergencies and impose involuntary hospitalization, restraints, isolation, and exclusion, as well as transfer to another service. All these create service-induced abandonment trauma (TA3) to the client. As a vicious cycle, the manifestation of self-induced traumas greatly intensify symptoms (1, 2, and 3) due to personality structure problems due to primary abandonment traumas (TA1). It further speeds up symptoms of impulsivity, anger, and self-harm behaviors (4, 5, 6, and 8).

In full-energy borderline condition, self-induced abandonment traumas together with service-induced abandonment traumas (TA2 + TA3) work together and intensify related symptoms (4, 5, 6, and 8) seriously. In some cases, it can last for many years. The manifestation of intensive impulsive, unstable, and self-harm symptoms exhausts clients' psychic, mental, and physical energies.

Individuals with BPD can also enter in a low-energy condition. Within this condition, symptoms due to personality structure problems (symptoms 1, 2, and 3) are still there but much subtler than before. Because of spontaneous abandonment by substituted attachment figures, abandonment fear greatly intensifies to a degree that hinders the manifestation of attachment hunger and abandonment anger.

Natures in the full-energy condition such as impulsivity, unstable affect, and self-harm symptoms decline accordingly. Instead, symptoms such chronic emptiness (symptom 7), paranoid ideation, and dissociative symptoms (symptom 9) prevail. In some cases, paranoid ideation can be intensified into psychotic episodes with prevailing but unclear paranoid delusions. Similarly, dissociative symptoms can also develop into dissociative disorders.

In the post-borderline condition, impulsivity, unstable affect, and self-harm behaviors were not there. Personality structure problems (symptoms 1, 2, and 3) are no longer sustained. Instead, chronic emptiness, paranoid ideation, and dissociative symptoms (symptoms 7 and 9) prevail and highly intensify.

Paranoid ideation is intensified and stabilized into paranoid schizophrenia. Chronic emptiness plus intense physical fatigue and loss of substituted attachment figures turn into a major depressive disorder. Dissociative symptoms with exhaustion of physical energy become prolonged and continuous dissociative disorders.

Co-morbidity of Drug Addiction and Borderline Personality Disorder

From related studies, Biskin and Paris (2013) concluded that 14.3% of those with alcohol abuse or dependence met the criteria for BPD, 16.8% of those dependent on cocaine received a diagnosis of BPD, and 18.5% of those who abused opioids met the criteria for BPD as well. However, some studies have noted that the averaged percentage of substance use is as high as 44.3 % (Biskin and Paris 2013). They concluded that

> About two-thirds of people with borderline disorder seriously abuse alcohol, street drugs, and/or prescribed drugs. This is a major factor that, if not corrected, contributes to poor treatment outcome of people with borderline disorder.
>
> Alcohol and drugs are often abused by people with borderline disorder to temporarily relieve the severe emotional pain that they experience, especially when under stress. Predictably, this relief is short lived. Even worse, the use of these substances markedly increases many of the symptoms of borderline disorder making substance abuse treatment all the more important. (Biskin and Parks 2013:45)

Drug Addiction and Borderline Personality Disorder: Interpretation and Intervention

Complexity of Borderline Personality Disorder and Drug Addiction

For people with BPD, many of them engage in substance abuse. Similarly, many people with substance abuse embrace borderline features. As mentioned in the previous chapter, there are several ways in which substance abuse and/or drug addiction are related with mental problems

1) Prolonged drug addiction leads to various types of mental illnesses.
2) Mental illness or problems are coped and delayed by spontaneous drug addiction.
3) Drug addiction goes together with various types of mental illnesses or problems.

In terms of BPD, it becomes the following:

1) Prolonged drug addiction leads to BPD.
2) Borderline conditions are coped and delayed by spontaneous drug addiction.
3) Drug addiction goes together with BPD.

For position 1, it is clear only 1B may be applicable to clients with borderline condition.

1B. Prolonged drug addiction nurtures drug-related interpersonal and psychosocial traumas that lead to occurrence of BPD.

As previously mentioned, most clinical research has shown that BPD is closely related to abandonment traumas and/or abuse in infancy, childhood, and adolescence. That means, prolonged drug addiction may not able to directly initiate the onset of borderline personality. However, for those clients with the pre-borderline condition, with abandonment trauma and/or abuse in infancy and childhood, their BPD in particular related symptoms in the full-energy condition may be speeded up by substance abuse. In fact, substance abuse is also counted as self-damaging behaviors in the symptoms of BPD. In chronic drug addiction, addiction-led traumas, such as being excluded and rejected by significant others, being labeled and stigmatized by members in the general public and members in the community, and impairment of social functioning, all of these exclusions, labeling, and stigmatizations are drug-led abandonment traumas. It certainly makes individuals feel dreadfully lonely, empty, and inferior.

For those individuals who do not have any borderline features before the onset of drug addiction, all these conditions certainly make individuals become self-isolated and excluded. On one hand, they eagerly want love and concern by others. On the other hand, they have no confidence in relating to others.

Given that they are addicted to drugs and they are labeled by others, they presume that all relationships with others, sooner or later, will end up with separation and abandonment. That means, they harbor a strong intimacy crisis that is quite similar to clients with borderline condition. The only difference is that they do not have outbursts of abandonment anger in the form of outward aggression as those clients in full borderline condition. Instead, abandonment anger may turn inward as self-harm or suicide because of being continuously excluded or rejected by others. They have a similar abandonment fear in which individuals are dreadfully afraid of being neglected and excluded by others.

They become very sensitive to others' comments and exclusions to a degree they prefer self-isolation or sticking to those drug-related peers in their daily life. In a more accurate term, as all these clients do not have primary abandonment traumas in their childhood as those with BPD, all these secondary abandonment traumas should be named "drug-led exclusion trauma."

Regarding position 2, BPD is delayed or can be coped with by drug addiction. It can be done in several ways.

2A. Drug addiction enables the individual to escape from the painfully oppressive reality, thus delayed onset of borderline personality disorder.
2B. Drug addiction provides a means for the individual to suppress and repress the recall and rebound of traumas that provoked BPD.
2C. Drug addiction alters the state of mind and body of the individual. At the same time, it also alters the individual's psychosocial and physical condition that leads to BPD.

For positions 2A and 2B, the oppressive reality for clients with BPD certainly is the primary and secondary abandonment traumas (TA1 and TA2). For clients with borderline condition, most of them harbor abandonment traumas by their caregivers in their infancy, childhood, and adolescence. As previously mentioned, the rebound of primary abandonment traumas make the individual suffer from the vicious cycle of attachment hunger, abandonment anger, abandonment fear, and intimacy crises. As a consequence, s/he is highly sensitive and overreacts to real or imagined abandonment in later life. In that condition drug addiction, in particular addiction to anesthetics and tranquilizers, may ease an individual's pains in facing the rebound of primary abandonment traumas. By doing so, the individual is less likely to engage in secondary (self-induced) abandonment traumas (TA2). That means, clients with pre-borderline condition may be less likely to move into the full-energy borderline condition, as self-induced traumas, abandonment anger, and fear are delayed by drug addiction. Whenever the memory of the abandonment trauma arrives, in particular the primary abandonment traumas is triggered, related negative emotions such as abandonment anger, fear, and chronic loneliness is also provoked. The individual engages in drug addiction to suppress or even repress all these memories and negative emotions.

Different types of drugs may have different effects in delaying the onset of BPD. Stimulants may give the individual extra courage and energy to engage in new relationships so that s/he can increase opportunities to find a substituted attachment figure. Once the substituted attachment figure is sought, the abandonment anger and fear are suppressed. The chronic loneliness is also temporarily covered. Tranquilizers help him/her to lower the intensity of negative emotions in the recall of abandonment traumas. Anesthetics help the client to detach from the painful reality of being abandoned by their significant others or substituted attachment figure.

2C. Drug addiction alters the state of mind and body of the individual. At the same time, it also alters the individual's psychosocial and physical condition that leads to BPD.

Drug addiction alters the state of mind and body in which the individual becomes physically weak with deterioration in the central nervous system, as well as in internal organs such as the liver, lungs, and kidneys. At the same time, the state mind is weakened by diffused consciousness continuously polluted by the ongoing drug addiction. The weak body and mind certainly make the individual feel incompetent in relating to others. At the same time, it also decreases others' interest in relating to them. The situation is closely related to position 1B (Prolonged drug addiction nurtures drug-related interpersonal and psychosocial traumas that leads to occurrence of BPD). In fact, in most cases, positions 2C and 1B reinforce one another. The weakening body and mind certainly reinforce various kinds of impairments in social functioning. It is understandable a client with chronic drug addiction, because of a weakened mind and body, gradually fails to continue his/her employment, to fulfill responsibility in the family, continue education, and to have normal relationships with his/her normal peers. All these further add to the labeling and stigmatization of being a drug addict. As a consequence, not only is s/he labeled and stigmatized by others but also feels isolated and rejected.

As mentioned in position 1B, all these are drug-led exclusion traumas. In other words, this type of trauma actually has two important components. One is being excluded by others, as drug addiction is morally and socially unaccepted by others. Another one is the physical and mental deterioration in which the client with chronic drug addiction feels inferior, inadequate, and shameful in relating to non-drug-related peers, family members, and friends. On one hand, s/he is addicted and severely dependent on drugs. On the other hand, s/he deeply realizes that the longer s/he is addicted to drugs, the more s/he is being rejected by others, and the more inferior and shameful and the weaker s/he is physically and mentally. In many cases, clients with chronic drug addiction are both addicted and obsessed with the drug. Being addictive means that s/he is totally dependent on drugs to ease out of his/her painful feelings in life, as well as in facing any adverse effects of drug addiction. Being obsessive means that s/he is fully aware of the negative effects of the drug. Together with this is an intense sense of guilt, shame, and reluctance in taking drugs. That means, in the process of drug addiction, the sense of addiction is intermingled with the sense of obsession. The individual has no way out. Despite feeling guilty, lonely, shameful, and reluctant in drug taking, s/he still needs to depend on drug addiction. Drug addiction is the only way to get rid of all these negative feelings. This is similar to a man who feels extremely thirsty in a boat in the rough sea. He needs to drink sea water to ease out of the sense of thirst. However, the more he drinks sea water, the more he feels thirsty.

All these drug-led exclusion traumas, together with the ambivalence and confusion of obsession and addiction, the individual is trapped within an intimacy crisis. On one hand, s/he feels dreadfully lonely and needs others' acceptance and togetherness. On the other hand, s/he feels shameful, too reluctant and too weak in relating with others. S/he is also highly sensitive to others' mild comments, slight rejections, and temporary separation.

Regarding position 3, drug addiction goes together with various types of mental illness or mental problems.

- 3A. Mental illnesses or problems occur before the intake of drug (mixing with the withdrawal effects of drugs).
- 3B. Mental illnesses or problems occur during the intake of drug (co-morbid with the stimulating effects of drugs).
- 3C. Mental illnesses or problems occur immediately after the intake of drugs (co-morbid with after the diminishing of the stimulating effects of drug).
- 3D. Mental illness or problems occur long after the intake of drugs.

For BPD, they become:

3A. Borderline personality disorder occurs before the intake of drugs (mixing with the withdrawal effects of drugs).
3B. Borderline personality disorder occurs during the intake of drug (co-morbid with the stimulating effects of drugs).
3C. Borderline personality disorder occurs immediately after the intake the drugs (co-morbid with after the diminishing of the stimulating effects of drugs).
3D. Borderline personality disorders occur long after the intake of drugs.

In position 3, position 3A occurs frequently. Positions 3B and 3C rarely exist in an actual situation. Position 3D is actually the same as position 2C. In fact, position 3A is the most common form in drug addiction. As previously mentioned, in the diagnosis of BPD, substance abuse is regarded as a symptom in self-damaging behavior.

The situation is particularly serious in female clients with chronic drug addiction. Many of them suffer from abandonment traumas in their childhood and adolescence. Because of this, they harbor a strong attachment need to have substituted attachment figures in their life. However, when they come close to all these substituted attachment figures, their unpleasant memories of being abandoned are triggered. Thus, they have an intimacy crisis in relating to others. On one hand, they have strong attachment hunger to substituted attachment figures. On the other hand, they harbor fear in intimate relationships. The intimacy crisis makes them fail to establish a suitable degree of intimacy with others. Also, any real or imagined separation from their substituted attachment figures may also arouse their abandonment anger in which they become highly sensitive, irritable, and overreactive to others' slight or mild criticism, ignorance, and non-attention. They easily reveal their anger and frustration. Some may even engage in emotional blackmailing of others by suicidal attempts, self-cutting, reckless driving, and other self-injurious behaviors. Facing all that, related substituted attachment figures may become highly frustrated and finally leave them, making them feel dreadfully lonely and empty. Under that sort of condition, individuals with BPD may easily regard drug addiction as the only substituted attachment figure to gratify their attachment hunger. For many female clients, they may attach to their boyfriends or spouses with chronic drug addiction. To affirm their attachment, they may engage in drug addiction together with their spouses or boyfriends. However, prolonged drug addiction also induces related traumas such as being abandoned by their family members or significant others, as they may crave drugs, with severe mental and physical deterioration. That means, on one hand, drug addiction serves as the final substituted attachment object. On the other hand, drug addiction alters the state of mind and body of the individual. At the same time, it also alters the individual's psychosocial and physical condition that leads to BPD. Chronic and severe drug addiction also induces further abandonment trauma that intensifies related symptoms, such as fluctuating emotions and relationship and self-image in BPD.

Case Illustration 1: Borderline Personality Disorder Occurs after Prolonged Drug Addiction

Combination of Positions 1B, 2C, and 3D

1B. Prolonged drug addiction nurtures drug-related interpersonal and psychosocial traumas that lead to occurrence of BPD.
2C. Drug addiction alters the state of mind and body of the individual. At the same time, it also alters the individual's psychosocial and physical condition that lead to BPD.
3D. Borderline personality disorders occur long after the intake of drugs.

Peter was a resident in a traditional village in Hong Kong. He had been engaged in the addiction of cough medicine for fifteen years. His ancestors had been living in this village for more than ten generations. His father was a prominent figure in the village. Members in this village regarded him as an informal leader who was familiar with every detail of related traditions and customs. His mother had died when Peter was only three years old. His father married another woman two years later. His stepmother gave birth to three daughters. Peter needed to help his stepmother in taking of his younger sisters.

All along, Peter was dreadfully busy. He had to take up the caring role of an eldest brother on one hand. On the other hand, he had to help his stepmother in taking up some household chores. At first, everything went well, as Peter could manage it well and was appreciated by his parents. Later, in secondary school life, Peter did not have time to study, and his academic performance was entirely unsatisfactory. He failed several subjects in Year 7. Instead of understanding his situation and helping him to ease out of his responsibility in the family, his father blamed Peter for his laziness in study. He physically punished Peter and urged for better results in the coming semester. This infuriated Peter. He felt very unfairly treated. He appeared to be very rebellious and refused to take care his younger sisters or do household chores. In no way could his father tolerate Peter's rebellion. He abused Peter by hitting him with a large and heavy stick. Peter fought with his father fiercely. Both of them were hurt after the fighting. Peter ran away and stayed outside with his classmates.

Despite his stepmother urging his father to say sorry, Peter refused to return home. From that time onward, Peter lived with his friends. In fact, all of them were delinquents. They introduced amphetamines to Peter. At first, Peter refused to do it. However, he was so depressed and frustrated about his father's abuse and maltreatment, he gradually accepted taking drugs as an effective means to release his frustration and tension in life. To earn a living, he also engaged in drug trafficking and selling. This made him rich, and he engaged with his girlfriend and they took drugs together.

At first, everything seemed fine and Peter enjoyed his life with money, his girlfriend, and drug sales and trafficking. After two years of frequent drug taking, Peter's physical and mental health deteriorated. He was no longer tactful and alert in doing his drug sale and trafficking. Unfortunately, he was caught by the police. He was charged with illegal drug trafficking and was sentenced for six months imprisonment. After this period, everyone left Peter, including his beloved girlfriend. He felt lonely, shameful, and in despair. When he was discharged, he tried to return home. His stepmother welcomed him back, but his father was furious about his immoral act in drug taking, drug sales, and drug trafficking. He even tried to hit Peter, saying that he would never regard Peter as his son. This made Peter feel severely shameful, angry, and inferior. He ran away again swearing that he would never return home.

He searched for a drug rehabilitation agency for help. The social worker there helped Peter look for job and a youth hostel for accommodation. At first, Peter worked well as a waiter in a Chinese restaurant. Nevertheless, being a waiter, in particular with the background as an ex-drug addict, was a tough life. His boss blamed him for trivial matters. It made Peter highly frustrated. Soon, Peter engaged in drug addiction again. He had frequent contacts with drug-related peers. Only a few of them got along again with Peter. Some committed suicide and some were caught by the police because of drug trafficking. Some went into drug detoxification centers. Peter felt dreadfully lonely.

Below is Peter's self-narration, demonstrating his chronic sense of loneliness and frustration.

Peter: This is certainly the darkest period of my life. Everybody has left me including my father, my stepmother, my previous girlfriend, and my former peers. Some committed suicide. Some went to drug detoxification centers. I have no friends, no relatives, and no one cares about me. My boss rejected me saying that I was nothing but a drug addict. I am empty, lonely, and a poor drug addict. I have even tried my best to quit it. No one believes in me. I am very lonely. Together with this loneliness is deep anger about why I was rejected by everyone.

When I was a child, I tried my best to take care of my stepsisters. I hated my father. He was so autocratic and unfair. Why did I have to do all the house chores while my stepmother and stepsisters enjoyed playing around? Why did my stepsisters behave wrongly yet I was the one to be punished? In fact, I tried my best my whole life. Even in drug sales and trafficking, I was always the one who sold the greatest amount of drugs to drug addicts. I was the most courageous one. The leader in the drug gang even said I had the best sales. For my girlfriend, I loved her deeply. I was willing to sacrifice everything including my life for her. However, she left me when I was in prison. She did not care about me anymore. When I got out of prison, I thought I could start a new life again, but everyone including my father and boss still firmly believed I was just a drug addict. I felt dreadfully lonely and inferior. I was angry with myself, my father, and my boss.

It was clear that Peter was very lonely, and he was spontaneously abandoned by his father, his girlfriend, and his peers. All these abandonment traumas were intolerable for him. He harbored severe abandonment anger toward his father, girlfriend, and peers. In fact, Peter was trapped within a dilemma of abandonment anger and fear. On one hand, he was angry with those who abandoned him. On the other hand, he harbored a strong urge to be accepted and cared by others. Under that condition, he was very sensitive to others' comments. Even with mild comments from others, he easily regarded that as being rejected and abandoned. As a consequence, even within an intense attachment hunger, he had a strong reluctance to relate to others. In other words, he had an intense and unbearable intimacy. Together with all these, he also had a highly fluctuating affect and uncontrollable anger. All these are main features of borderline condition. Apart from these, Peter also had a chronic sense of emptiness. That means, for Peter, his prolonged drug addiction nurtured drug-related interpersonal and psychosocial traumas, in particular abandonment traumas that led to the occurrence of borderline features (position 1B). In the same ways, drug addiction altered Peter's state of mind and body and psychosocial condition that led to borderline condition (position 2C). He became more and more unstable emotionally and mentally. His body and physical conditions deteriorated accordingly. Within all these poor mental and physical conditions, he felt more and more inferior and fearful in connecting with others. Despite him desperately seeking others' concern, his poor mental and physical condition deterred him from relating to others and increased his attachment hunger and intimacy crisis in relating with others. As a consequence, borderline disorder occurs long after the intake of drugs for Peter (3D).

Case Illustration 2: Borderline Personality Disorder Occurs Before Drug Addiction (3A)

Mary was born in a happy family in which her father was a senior teacher in a primary school. Her mother was a senior clerk in a big shipping company. Her parents loved her deeply, and she was happy and contented. Every Sunday, her parents took her swimming at the beach. Her father was well educated and encouraged Mary to enjoy watching movies, operas, and Chinese operas. Unfortunately, the happy life came to an end when Mary was five years old. Her father committed adultery with his colleague in the office. Mary's mother was furious. She had a severe quarrel with her husband and threatened him to leave this woman immediately by resigning his job. The next day, her father ran away and never returned.

From that time onward, Mary's life was miserable. Mary's mother suffered from severe depression. In no way could she take good care of little Mary under the influence of severe depressive mood. Little Mary was under the care of her grandmother who was very old. All she could provide merely was minimal physical care and safety. Mary was lonely and anxious all along. She urged others for love and care, but she could not get it in her childhood. She never forgot a scene at five years old in kindergarten.

There was a heavy rainfall in which all students were escorted home by their parents. She was the last one in kindergarten waiting for her grandmother to take her home. Finally, her grandmother came. Mary felt deeply frustrated. She had a temper tantrum. She rushed into the heavy rainfall refusing to take the umbrella. Her grandmother was very angry and used another umbrella to hit her. Mary cried bitterly. She then suffered from a high fever for two weeks.

After that, her grandmother refused to take care of her and transferred her back to her mother. At that time, her mother was in a better mood. Her mood had lightened. She took care of Mary, accompanied her to school, and helped her to finish her homework assignments. Under her mother's care, Mary's emotions stabilized. She was lovely and clever. Mary's kindergarten life was happy and enjoyable.

Unfortunately, when Mary was ten years old, her mother married another man. He was initially a rich merchant. At first, her stepfather got along with Mary well. Later, his business was ruined, and he was bankrupted. From that time onward, he became an alcoholic. Whenever he was drunk, he abused both Mary and her mother. Mary was angry with him. She fought with him during the abuse with a result of more severe physical abuse being imposed.

In Year 10, Mary ran away from home. She could tolerate no more. She cohabitated with her boyfriend who was a delinquent and engaged in drug trafficking. From that time onward, Mary began to abuse

> amphetamines with her boyfriend. She also helped her boyfriend to engage in drug trafficking and sales.

It was clear that Mary suffered from frequent abandonment from her significant others. All these were abandonment traumas (AT) that nurtured a borderline condition. First, her father committed adultery with his colleague in his office and ran away (AT1). Second, since her mother suffered from severe depression, Mary was separated from her (AT2) and was taken care of by her old grandmother who could only provide minimal physical care. Unfortunately, she could not take good care of her and left her uncared for on a rainy day that was certainly a traumatic experience for little Mary (AT3). Later, she was then abandoned by her and transferred back to her mother (AT4). At first, her mother treated her well, but later she married again and her husband was bankrupt several years later and began to physically abuse Mary (AT5). It was at that time in which frequent and prolonged abandonment trauma nurtured and provoked Mary's onset of BPD. Below is Mary's mother description of Mary's pathological condition at that time.

> Mary's mother: At that time, Mary was in Year 9, and my husband was bankrupt. He was frustrated by this. He could not accept the fact that he had lost everything, including his business, which he had built up over decade by resolving numerous difficulties, his reputation, and respect among his peers. He was severely depressed and addicted to alcohol. Day-and-night drinking was the only means for him to escape from all this frustration. Whenever he was drunk, he was very confused and angry. Any disturbance from us would provoke his aggressiveness, and he abused us physically.
>
> Mary was the one who suffered a lot from his physical abuse. He tried to smash her with anything nearby, such as a chair, clothes hanger, stick, or brush. This was highly humiliating and harmful to Mary. At first, she tried to escape from the abuse. He restrained and restricted her from running away. Mary screamed and fought back. However, the more she did so, the more furious my husband became. Once, Mary was seriously hurt from his abuse and needed three days hospitalization. From that time onward, Mary's emotions became highly unstable. She was easily

provoked by any comment from others. She easily broke into intense anger. She cursed others seriously. I had seen her twice cutting her wrists in her bed with intense crying.

She also engaged in courtship. She fell in love with a male classmate at school. She attached to him deeply and demanded his prolonged presence and togetherness in any moment. At first, he enjoyed it, feeling that Mary loved him deeply. Later, he was intolerable with Mary's endless demands. They separated. Mary was deeply depressed and sad. She cut her wrist deeply. I told her to be rational and sensible. She was furious. She cursed me that I was the black sheep of the family. I was the one bringing misfortunes and sufferings to her. I cursed her back. She ran away. From that time, she never returned home.

From Mary's mother description, it was clear that Mary suffered from BPD. She manifested a strong attachment hunger to his boyfriend. She committed self-damaging behavior in a form self-cutting and suicide gestures. She harbored uncontrollable affect and outbursts of anger. She was also highly sensitive to the real or imagined abandonment from her parents as well as from her boyfriend. All this clearly showed that Mary suffered from BPD.

Mary ran away and cohabited with her boyfriend who was a delinquent. He engaged in drug trafficking and sales. They also took amphetamines together. However, their relationship did not last long. Two years later, her boyfriend was caught by the police and imprisoned. Mary felt lonely and sad for the loss of her boyfriend. She took a high dosage of amphetamines and intended to commit suicide in the railway. Fortunately, she was restrained by her friends. She was faint near the railway line and was taken to a nearby hospital. She stayed there for two weeks.

Later, she worked as a waitress in a Chinese restaurant. She then got along with another boyfriend who was a waiter in this restaurant. They liked each other, and at first their relationship was fine. Later, Mary was pregnant. However, her boyfriend was afraid to take a parental role, and Mary was very angry. She left her boyfriend and had an abortion. She was very frustrated and began to take drugs again. This time, she took ketamines with her drug-related peers.

From that time onward, Mary no longer believed in a permanent courtship and love. Instead, she engaged in frequent causal sex and drug addiction with her numerous boyfriends or sex partners. Ketamines, amphetamines, or tranquilizers became the gateway to chronic drug and sex addiction. It was clear that sex and drugs became Mary's substituted attachment in facing prolonged loneliness, emptiness, and abandonment by her parents, boyfriends, and other peers.

The more Mary was engaged in drug addiction and sex addiction, her health and mental condition deteriorated drastically. Prolonged usage of ketamines damaged her bladder and liver. She was weak and had to urinate every half hour. She also had a liver infection. Under this condition, Mary sought help from a social worker in a drug addiction and rehabilitation center. The social worker, Michelle, advised Mary to have drug detoxification in a detoxification village.

Mary stayed there for two months and successfully abstained from drug addiction. While Mary could have a new life, she came down with a high fever for two weeks with other symptoms. The medical practitioners advised Mary to have an HIV test. Unfortunately, the test result showed that she was HIV positive. Mary was totally shocked by this bad news. On one hand, she knew that it was the consequence of the unsafe sex and sex addiction. On the other hand, she felt it was dreadfully unfair, as she was already abandoned by her parents and her boyfriends.

From Mary's case, it clearly shows that conditions in clients with BPD and drug addiction are highly complicated and ambivalent. The situation is particularly serious for those who have onset of BPD long before drug addiction. There are several complications that commonly occur in clients.

1) Drug addiction is used as a substitute attachment in facing prolonged loneliness and attachment fear in frequent losses of primary attachment figures (being abused, separated, rejected, or abandoned by parents, grandparents, and close relatives who had taken care of the client in early life or current life), or substituted attachment figures (being abused, rejected, or separated by boyfriends, girlfriends, or peers).
2) Drug addiction is used as a means to suppress or reject inner pain in facing frequent abandonment traumas and other current sufferings and hardships in life.

3) Drug addiction is used as a means to release abandonment anger by inducing self-harm to one's body and mind through drug addiction.
4) Drug addiction as a means to attach to substituted attachment figures such as boyfriends, girlfriends, or peers by taking drugs together.

It is clear in Mary's case that drug addiction was used as a means to cope with the manifestation of BPD. However, as time went by, prolonged drug addiction also increased the severity of her borderline condition by inducing drug-related abandonment traumas. That means, the more prolonged and severe the drug addiction is, the more excluded, rejected, and devaluated the client is by their substituted attachment figure. First, the client's mental and physical health condition is worsened by the chronic drug addiction. Second, the client is also labeled as a drug addict and substance abuser and is thus frequently excluded, labeled, and belittled by significant others, such as family members, close peers, colleagues, and employers.

Complications of Borderline Personality Disorder, Trauma, and Drug Addiction

As mentioned in chapter 1, drug addiction and traumas intermingle each other in a complicated way. On one hand, drug addiction provides a temporary coping and escape for individuals to face traumas, sufferings, and hardships in life and delay the onset of possible mental problems (Force A). On the other hand, prolonged drug addiction provokes and induces related traumas and imposes physical and mental harm that nurtures the occurrence of severe mental illness (Force B).

There are four ways in which these two forces interact with one another. They can be listed as follows:

1) Force A inhibits Force B.
2) Force B inhibits Force A.
3) Force A reinforces Force B.
4) Force A combines Force B.

In cases of clients with borderline personality disorders, related traumas are abandonment trauma. That means, drug addiction is used as coping for abandonment trauma on one hand (Force A). On the other hand, drug addiction can also induce further abandonment trauma (Force B).

All these four combinations occur within the process of drug addiction in the following state.

Stage 1: Force A Only (Initial or Occasional Users)

In this stage, Force B is too early to occur (when the individual attempts drug addiction and uses it occasionally). In clients with BPD, Force A means drug addiction can be used to cope with abandonment trauma. Force B (drug addiction can induce further abandonment trauma) does not occur. Individuals suffer from prevailing abandonment traumas in their developmental process. They may harbor intensive attachment hunger together with abandonment anger and fear in relating to others in which symptoms of BPD are provoked. However, drug addiction is used as a means to delay or inhibit the occurrence of the BPD. First, drug addiction can be served a substitute attachment object. Second, drug addiction is used as a means to attach to drug-related peers, in particular sex or courtship partners. Third, drug addiction is used as a means to absorb or ventilate abandonment anger and fear. Fourth, drug addiction is regarded as a way of self-harm so as to punish those primary and substituted attachment figures that abandon the clients.

Stage 2: Force A Inhibits Force B (Regular Users: Initial Addiction)

As previously mentioned, Force B begins to occur as the individual has taken drugs for a period of time, usually one or two months. Related adverse and harmful effects are still mild and within an acceptable level. The individual uses drugs regularly to cope with his/her life stress, frustration, and trauma. For clients in the borderline condition, they are used to taking drug to delay the onset of BPD. In doing so, the harmful and adverse effects begin to evolve. It can be psychological and physical dependence and withdrawal effects. All these hinder clients' actualizations of their attachment hunger toward normal peers and relatives. Instead, they tend to attach to drug-related peers, and their regular drug addiction makes them begin to become unacceptable to normal peers and relatives. That means the deteriorating effects of Force B on physical, mental and social conditions begin to appear. Clients begin to have initial abandonment traumas.

Stage 3: Force A Combines with Force B (Long-Term Regular Users: Full Addiction)

As mentioned in the previous chapter, in Stage 3, Force B begins to prevail, resulting in significant physical and mental damage for the individual. Related damages are still tolerable and acceptable for the individual. S/he fully enjoys the drug addiction. S/he is fully involved in the smoothly and paralyzing effect of the drug. Thus, s/he enjoys the effect of drug taking on one hand and is aware of the serious damage in the future on the other hand.

S/he feels a bit confused and ambivalent, in particular within the addictive process. In clients with BPD, clients' abandonment traumas created by drugs begin to prevail. This can be deteriorating health that may hinder clients' employment abilities. Prolonged drug addiction that is being rejected by family members as well former friends and peers. This can also be abandonment traumas by primary or substituted attachment figures who abandon the client because of drug addiction. The individual is circled by drug-related peers only.

However, all these are still tolerable to the clients. S/he uses close attachment to drug-related peers to replace the gradual abandonment by family members and friends. She uses the stimulating or tranquilizing effects of drugs to lessen the abandonment anger and fear. The situation is getting worse but still at a tolerable level.

S/he seems to have no way but only engaging in this gradually deteriorating situation. The pain from developmental abandonment trauma by primary attachment figures and separation from substituted attachment figures is intensified by the drug-induced abandonment trauma. However, the individual can only rely on further drug addiction to ease out of all these growing pains. S/he has no way out except waiting for the rock bottom of drug addiction.

Stage 4: Force A Reinforces Force B (Chronic Addiction)

In Stage 4, Force A reinforces Force B. Related physical and mental damage to clients with drug addiction are very significant and substantial to a degree that their normal ego functioning and social functioning are hindered. It can be problems in employment, education, and normal daily interaction and living pattern. Related clients are fully aware that continuous drug addiction could result in severe damage physically, mentally, psychologically, and socially. However, they do not have any way out. They can only cope with that sort of fear and worry by even more intensive and frequent drug addiction. Deep down in their minds, they know that one day they will totally collapse both mentally and physically. Together with the total rejection from their friends and relatives before chronic drug addiction. Even when they approach them, they try to avoid them. They feel shameful and dreadfully inferior to see them. The only way they approach them is for money to buy drugs. For clients with BPD, at this stage, most of them have low-energy borderline personality features in which abandonment fear is far more intensive than abandonment anger. They tend to isolate themselves rather than having strong attachment hunger to approach and attach to others. Their intensive abandonment anger turns inward and becomes severe depression, anxiety, and psychosomatic symptoms. They feel both shameful and guilty about themselves. Many of them engage in spontaneous self-harm or even suicidal gestures to end their life. However, the tranquilizing, stimulating effects of drugs may help them to alleviate their inner pain and reduce the onset of all these acts of self-harm and suicide. Many clients at this stage, with some very mild support from others or related social welfare agencies, can maintain their chronic stage for a long period of time.

Stage 5: Force B Inhibits Force A (Rock Bottom of Chronic Addiction)

Force B inhibits Force A implies the rock bottom of chronic drug addiction. As previously mentioned, related clients are in the lowest ebb of his/her life with severe poverty, unemployment, being abused, oppression, and victimization. They have nowhere to go. Their health is deteriorating, and many of them are facing the final days of total failure of their kidneys, bladder, liver, or other severe physical disease. Deep down in their mind, they are fully aware that only immediate detoxification can save them from the accumulated harmful effects of drug addiction. But they do not have enough courage, determination, resources, or support to do so. All they can do is give in to the continuous craving for drugs until the final day comes. In the borderline condition, the client's dissociative symptoms increase intensely with deteriorating health conditions. They are dreadfully lonely, fearful, regretful, and shameful in meeting and relating. An extreme sense of chronic emptiness, together with prevailing paranoid ideation, dissociative symptoms, and depressive mood, may turn the client into a post-borderline condition. Many may finally harbor severe mental illness, such as schizophrenia, major depressive disorder, or severe dissociative disorders.

Conclusion

This chapter is a comprehensive discussion about drug addiction and BPD. The writer begins with a full articulation of the etiology of BPD as well as various borderline conditions, including pre-borderline, full-energy borderline, low-energy borderline, and post-borderline condition. There are also various positions between drug addiction and BPD. The first is prolonged drug addiction leading to borderline condition. The second is borderline condition coped with or delayed by drug addiction. The third is drug addiction going together with borderline conditions. Finally, various combinations of Force A and Force B in drug addiction are discussed. All these have strong implications in working with clients with co-morbid drug addiction and borderline features. In various conditions and combinations, related intervention should be highly different. For example, in low-energy borderline condition and chronic addiction, related professionals should focus more on the client's deteriorating health problems, self-isolation, and dissociative symptoms. Apart from detoxification and harm reduction, it is important to improve the client's health condition, cure related dissociative symptoms, and increase the client's social interaction and relationship with healthy peers, family members, and significant others.

Chapter 4

UNDERSTANDING AND INTERVENTION FOR PEOPLE WITH DRUG ADDICTION OPPRESSION, ABUSE, AND PSYCHOSIS

INTRODUCTION

In this chapter, the writer attempts to have a comprehensive interpretation of psychosis and chronic drug addiction. Related literature shows that chronic drug addiction is closely related to the onset of schizophrenia or vice versa. People with chronic drug addiction are vulnerable to the onset of schizophrenia, in particular those addicted to amphetamines, hallucinogens, and ketamines. This chapter begins with the diagnosis and etiology of schizophrenia, co-morbidity of schizophrenia, and drug addiction. Then various positions of drug addiction and schizophrenia are mentioned. Force A and Force B combinations are discussed. Their implications to clinical practice are also figured out.

DIAGNOSIS, ETIOLOGY OF SCHIZOPHRENIA

Diagnosis from DSM IV and DSM V

There is a change of schizophrenia from DSM IV (APA 1994) to DSM V (APA 2013). That can be described and compared in the following Table 1.

Table 4. The Clinical Profile from DSM IV and DSM V

DSM IV	DSM V
A. Characteristic symptoms: Two (or more) of the following, each present for a significant portion of time during a one-month period (or less if successfully treated) 1. Delusion 2. Hallucination 3. Disorganized speech 4. Grossly disorganized or catatonic behavior 5. Negative symptoms, i.e., affecting flattening, alogia or avolition *Note: Only one criterion A symptom is required if delusions are bizarre or hallucinations consist of a voice keeping u a running commentary on the persons' behaviour or thoughts, or two or more voices conversing with each other*	**A.** Two (or more) of the following, each present for a significant portion of time during a one-month period (or less if successfully treated). **At least one of these must be 1, 2, or 3** 1. Delusion 2. Hallucination 3. Disorganized speech (e.g., frequent derailment or incoherence) 4. Grossly disorganized or catatonia behavior) 5. Negative symptom (i.e., diminished emotional expression or avolition)
B. Social/ occupational dysfunction For a significant portion of the time since the onset of the disturbance, on or more major areas of functioning such as work, interpersonal relations, or self-care are markedly below the level achieved prior to the onset (or when the onset is in childhood or adolescence, failure to achieve expected level of interpersonal, academic or occupational achievement)	B. Social/ occupational dysfunction For a significant portion of the time since the onset of the disturbance, on or more major areas of functioning such as work, interpersonal relations, or self-care are markedly below the level achieved prior to the onset (or when the onset is in childhood or adolescence, there is failure to achieve expected level of interpersonal, academic or occupational achievement)

DSM IV	DSM V
C. Duration Continuous signs of the disturbance persist for at least 6 months. This 6 month period must include in at least 1 month of symptoms (or less if successfully treated) that meet criterion A (i.e., Active phase symptoms) and may include periods of prodromal or residual symptoms. During these prodromal or residual periods, the signs of the disturbance may be manifested by only negative symptoms or two or more symptoms listed in criterion A present in attenuated form (e.g., Odd beliefs, unusual perceptual experiences) D. Schizoaffective and Mood Disorder Exclusion E. Substance/general medical examination exclusion F. Relationship to a pervasive developmental disorder Classification of longitudinal course (can be applied only after at least one year has elapsed since the initial onset of active phase symptoms) Episode with Interepisode residual symptoms With prominent negative symptoms Episode with no Interepisode residual symptoms Continuous with prominent negative symptoms Single Episode in Partial Remission with Prominent negative symptoms Single Episode in Full Remission Other or Unspecified Pattern	C. Duration Continuous signs of the disturbance persist for at least 6 months. This 6 month period must include in at least 1 month of symptoms (or less if successfully treated) that meet criterion A (i.e., Active phase symptoms) and may include periods of prodromal or residual symptoms. During these prodromal or residual periods, the signs of the disturbance may be manifested by only negative symptoms or two or more symptoms listed in criterion A present in attenuated form (e.g., Odd beliefs, unusual perceptual experiences) D. Schizoaffective and Mood Disorder Exclusion E. Substance/general medical examination exclusion F. Relationship to a pervasive developmental disorder Classification of longitudinal course (can be applied only after at least one year has elapsed since the initial onset of active phase symptoms) **Specify if:** 1. **First Episode, currently in acute episode** (First manifestation of the disorder meeting the defining diagnostic symptoms and time criteria. An acute episode is a time period in which the symptom criteria are fulfilled. 2. **First Episode, currently in partial remission:** Partial remission is a period of time during which an improvement after a previous episode is maintained and in which the defining criteria of the disorder are only partially fulfilled. 3. **First Episode, currently in full remission**: Full remission is a period of time after a previous episode during which no disorder specific symptoms are present. 4. **Multiple Episode, currently in partial remission**

Table 4. (Continued)

DSM IV	DSM V
	5. Multiple Episode, currently in full remission 6. Continuous: Symptoms fulfilling the diagnostic symptom criteria of the disorder are remaining for the majority of the illness course, with subthreshold symptoms periods being very brief relative to the overall course. **Specify if:** **With Catatonia** **Specify current severity:** Severity is rated by a quantitative assessment of the primary symptoms of psychosis, including delusions, hallucinations, disorganized speech, abnormal psychomotor behavior, and negative symptoms. Each of these symptoms may be rated for its current severity (most severe in the last 7 days) on a 5 point scale ranging from 0 to 4.

Highlights of Changes from DSM IV to DSM V Schizophrenia Spectrum and Other Psychotic Disorders

Two changes were made to Criterion A for schizophrenia:

1) The elimination of the special attribution of bizarre delusion and Schneiderian first-rank auditory hallucinations (e.g., two or more voices conversion) leading to the requirement that at least two Criterion A symptoms for any diagnosis of schizophrenia. And
2) The addition of the requirement that at least one of the Criterion A symptoms must be delusions, hallucinations, or disorganized speech.

The DSM IV subtypes of schizophrenia were eliminated due their limited diagnostic stability, low reliability, and poor validity. Instead, a dimensional approach to rating severity of the core symptoms of schizophrenia is included in DSM V Section III to capture the important heterogeneity in symptom type and severity expressed across individuals with psychotic disorders. Schizoaffective disorder is reconceptualized as a longitudinal instead of a cross-sectional diagnosis—more comparable to schizophrenia, bipolar disorder, and major depressive disorder, which are bridged by this condition—and required that a major mood episode be present for a majority of the total disorder's duration for Criterion A has been met. Criterion A for delusional disorder no longer has the requirement that the delusions must be non-bizarre; a specifier is now included for bizarre-type delusions to provide continuity with DSM IV. Criteria for catatonia are described uniformly across DSM V. Furthermore, catatonia may be diagnosed with a specifier (for depressive, bipolar, and psychotic disorder, including schizophrenia), in the context of a known medical conditions, or as other specified diagnoses. (APA 2013: 810)

Etiology

From the symptoms listed in DSM IV, there are three main groups of symptoms. They are positive symptoms, negative symptoms, and the first-rank symptoms. Positive symptoms include delusion, hallucination, catatonia, and disorganized speech. Negative symptoms include alogia, avolition, anhedonia, and blunted affect. First-rank symptoms are thought insertion, thought broadcasting, and two voices arguing with one another. In clinical diagnosis, delusions and hallucinations are the most explicit positive symptoms in people with schizophrenia.

Positive Symptoms

According to DSM IV, delusions are erroneous beliefs or misinterpretation of perceptions:

> Delusions are erroneous beliefs that usually involve a misinterpretation of perceptions or experiences. Their content may include a variety of theme (e.g., Persecutory, referential, somatic, religious, or grandiose)... The distinction between a delusion and a strongly held idea is sometimes difficult to make and depends on the degree of conviction with which the belief is held despite clear contradictory evidence… Delusions are deemed bizarre if they are clearly implausible and not understandable and do not derive from ordinary life experience. … Delusion that expresses a loss of control over mind or body (those included among Schneider's first-rank symptoms) are generally considered to be bizarre... thought withdrawal (taken by others)... thought insertion (thought input by others) ... delusion of control (mind or body control by outside force) (APA 1994: 275)

According to the preceding definitions, delusions should consist of the following components:

1) Erroneous belief
2) Misinterpretation of perceptions or experiences
3) Various themes in contents (persecutory, referential, somatic, religious, or grandiose)
4) Hard to distinction between delusions and strongly held idea

First-Rank Symptoms

Once the delusions are bizarre, they are classified as first-rank symptoms. In terms of self-fragmentation, bizarre delusions are more severe than positive symptoms.

Hallucination is defined by DSM IV as follows:

> Hallucination may occur in any sensory modality (e.g., auditory, visual, olfactory, gustatory, and tactile, auditory hallucinations are by far the most common and characteristic of schizophrenia. Auditory hallucinations are usually experienced as voices, whether familiar or unfamiliar, that are perceived as distinct from the person's own thoughts.

> The content may be quite variable, although pejorative or threatening voices are especially common. Certain types of auditory hallucinations (i.e., two or more voices conversing with one another or voices maintaining a running commentary on the person's thought or behavior) have been considered to be particularly characteristic of schizophrenia and were included among Schneider's list of first-rank symptoms. If these types of hallucinations are present, then only this single symptom is needed to satisfy Criterion A. (American Psychiatric Association 1994: 275)

In other words, hallucinations consist of the following characteristics:

a) As a sensory modality (auditory, visual, olfactory, gustatory, tactile)
b) Auditory one is the most common one
c) It can be a familiar or unfamiliar voice
d) It is distinct from one's thought

The preceding definitions on delusion and hallucination clearly show that that is not a clear distinction between strongly held ideas and delusion, and between oversensitive perception and hallucination. Also, both definitions do not provide a description of linkage of reality. It tends to presumes that people with schizophrenia embrace a faulty interpretation, belief, and perception of reality.

Disorganized thinking, according to DSM IV is interpreted as follows:

> Disorganized thinking (formal thought disorder, "loosening of association" has been argued by some (Bleuler, in particular) to be the single most important features of Schizophrenia because of the difficulty inherent in developing and objective definition of "thought disorder" and because in a clinical setting inference about thought are based primarily on individual's speech, the concept of disorganized speech... Because mildly disorganized speech is common and nonspecific, the symptom must be severe enough to substantially impair effective communication (American Psychiatric Association 1994: 276)

Disorganized thinking according to DSM IV consists of the following:

1) Loosening of association
2) Based on clients' speech
3) Impairment in effective communication.

Again, the definition of disorganized thinking is hard to make clear. As mildly disorganized speech is common and nonspecific, it is quite hard for related professionals to have a clear diagnosis in this area. In fact, clinically speaking, related professionals may fail to have a clear and precise picture of positive symptoms in terms of delusions, hallucinations, catatonia, and disorganized speech. Very often, psychosis and insanity is defined by its consequence rather than by its actual features. Thus, in criterion B, all clients with psychosis should have a marked impairment in psychosocial functioning. It can be problems and difficulties in employment, family life, and communication with others. In some severe cases, there can be severe problems in personal hygiene and highly confused mental state (Yip 2018).

Negative Symptoms

According to Andreasen (1984), negative symptoms of schizophrenia are defined as the lack of important abilities including alogia, affective flattening, avolition, and anhedonia. Andreasen developed the (1984) Scale for the Assessment of Negative Symptoms (SANS). Alogia means poverty of speech. It contains deficits in speech fluency, and blocked thoughts, as well as short and empty replies to questions. Andreasen (1984) in her SANS describes alogia as follows:

> Alogia is a general term coined to refer to the impoverished thinking and cognition that often occur in subjects with schizophrenia (Greek *a* = none; *logos* = mind, thought). Subjects with alogia have thinking processes that seem empty, turgid or slow. Since thinking cannot be observed directly, it is inferred from subject's speech. The two major manifestations of alogia are nonfluent empty speech (poverty of speech) and fluent empty speech (poverty of content of speech). Blocking and increased latency or response may also reflect alogia. (Andreasen 1984: 5)

For assessment, it consists of the following components:

1) Poverty of speech (Brief, concrete, unelaborated, monosyllabic or even unanswered replies to questions)
2) Poverty of content of speech (Vague, over-abstracted, over-concrete, repetitive and stereotyped speech.)
3) Blocking (Interruption of a trained speech before a thought or idea has been completed)
4) Increased Latency of Response (Take a long time to reply to questions than is usually considered normal) (Andreasen 1984: 5–7)

Avolition is the reduction, difficulty, or inability of persons with schizophrenia to initiate and persist in goal-directed behavior. For example, persons with schizophrenia are no longer interested in going out and meeting with friends or show enthusiasm. They are no longer interested in much of anything, sitting in the house for many hours a day doing nothing (Schizophrenia.com 2004).

Andreason (1984) defines avolition as:

> Avolition manifests itself as a characteristic lack of energy, drive and interest. Subjects are unable to mobilize themselves to initiate or persist in completing many different kinds of tasks. Unlike the diminishing energy or interest of depression, the avolition symptom complex in schizophrenia is usually not accompanied by saddened or depressed affect. The avolition symptom complex often leads to severe social and economic impairment (Andreason 1984: 7)

That means, avolition is a state of physical and mental fatigue, in which the individual has no interest or energy to do anything. It consists of the following components in assessing symptoms of avolition:

1) Poor Grooming and Personal Hygiene (Infrequent grooming, bath, dirty hands, soiled clothing.)
2) Impersistence at Work or School (Absence, infrequency in attending school and work)

3) Physical Anergia (Physically inert, sitting at home and doing nothing and poor participation in any activities)

(Andreasen 1984: 7–8)

In psychology, anhedonia is an inability to experience pleasure from normally pleasurable life events, such as eating, exercise, and social or sexual interaction. Anhedonia is also regarded as an important negative symptom commonly seen in persons with schizophrenia, schizoaffective disorder, schizoid personality disorder, and other mental disorders (Schizophrenia.com 2004). Andreasen (1984) defines anhedonia as a state of asociality.

> This symptom complex encompasses the schizophrenic subject's difficulties in experiencing interests or pleasure. It may express itself as a loss of interest in pleasurable activities, an inability to experience pleasure when participating in activities normally considered pleasurable, or a lack of involvement in social relationship of various kinds. (Andreasen 1984: 9)

It consists of the following components in assessing the state of anhedonia:

1) Few or no recreational interest or activities (ranging from few or no hobbies, to loss of interest in passive activities, such as watching TV, and finally to complete and intractable inability to become involved or enjoy activities)
2) Decrement in sexual interest and activities (loss of activities in sexual intercourse)
3) Inability to feel intimacy and closeness
4) Restricted and poor relationship with friends and peers of either sex

(Andreasen 1984: 9–10)

Affective flattening is the reduction in the range and intensity of emotional expression, including facial expression, voice tone, and eye. Persons with schizophrenia have problems in interpreting body language or using appropriate body language in the expression of their feelings and cognition. In SANS, affective flattening is defined as follows:

> Affective flattening or blunting manifests itself is a characteristic impoverishment of emotional expression, reactivity, and feeling. It can be evaluated by observation of the subject's behavior and responsiveness during a routine interview. The rating of some items may be affected by drugs, since the Parkinsonian side effect of phenothiazines may lead to make-like faces and diminished associated movement. Other aspects of affect such as responsivity or appropriateness will not be affected, however (Andreason 1984: 2)

In SANS, it consists of the following components:

1) Unchanging Facial Expression (The subject appears wooden, mechanical, frozen)
2) Decreased Spontaneous Movement (The subject sits quietly throughout the interview and shows few or no spontaneous body movements)
3) Paucity of Expressive Gestures (The subject does not use his body as an aid in experience his ideas)
4) Poor Eye Contact (The subject avoids looking at others or using his eyes as an aid in expression. He appears to be staring into space even when he is talking)
5) Affective Non-Responsivity (Failure to simile or laugh when prompted may be tested by smiling or joking)
6) Lack of Vocal Inflections (Speech has a monotonic quality, and important words are not emphasized through changes in pitch or volume)
7) Inappropriate Affect (Affect expressed is inappropriate or incongruous, not simply flat or blunted. Most typically, this manifestation of affective disturbance takes the form of smiling or assuming a silly facial expression.)

(Andreason 1984: 2–3)

Apart from avolition, anhedonia, affect blunting, and alogia, attention in schizophrenia is also poor and inadequate.

> Attention is often poor in schizophrenics. The subject may have trouble focusing his attention, or he may only be able to focus sporadically and erratically. He may ignore attempts to converse with him, wander away while in the middle of an activity or take, or appear to be inattentive when engaged in formal testing or interviewing. He may or may not be aware of his difficulty in focusing his attention... Inattentiveness appears in social situation or activities... He looks uninvolved or unengaged in conservation... poor concentration when playing games, reading and watching TV. (Andreasen 1984: 11)

Co-morbidity of Drug Addiction and Schizophrenia

Prevalence

Co-morbidity of drug addiction and schizophrenia can be understood in two ways. One is the prevalence of clients with psychosis that take substances or engage in drug addiction to deal with their psychotic symptoms.

Another one is prevalence of substance-induced psychosis in which prolonged substance abuse leads to the onset of psychosis. The Caton et al. (2005) study showed the following results.

> The study is based on a referred sample of 400 subjects interviewed at baseline. Participants had at least 1 psychotic symptom assessed during administration of the research protocol, had used alcohol and/or other drugs within the past 30 days, and had no psychiatric inpatient history before the past 6 months. Overall, 169 (44%) were diagnosed as having substance-induced psychosis and 217 (56%) as having primary psychosis. (Caton et al. 2005: 45)

Dual diagnosis is a usual term in describing the concurrence of drug addiction and schizophrenia and other mental illnesses.

Reasons for Substance Abuse by People with Schizophrenia

Smith and Hucker (1993), based on a comprehensive review of related studies, concluded that there are several reasons for substance abuse by people with schizophrenia.

First, those clients with better premorbid adjustment are more sociable and therefore exposed to more opportunities to experiment with illicit drugs and alcohol. Second, after the onset of the schizophrenic psychosis, the substance abuse accelerates in an attempt to cope with the stress associated with the illness. Third, being a drug addict or substance abuser is a better self-identity than being a mental patient in social interaction in certain subcultures. Fourth, the effect of substance abuse can mediate symptoms of schizophrenia. Psychostimulant drugs may reduce negative symptoms such as apathy and withdrawal, whereas alcohol and benzodiazepines can temporarily suppress psychotic symptoms; a possibility is that psychostimulant drugs counteract distressing neuroleptic-induced extrapyramidal side effects, particularly akathisia.

Substance-Induced Psychosis

Psychosocial Causes and Controversies

Smith and Hucker (1993), according to related studies, also affirm that there is heavy premorbid consumption of alcohol and illicit drugs in individuals who later become schizophrenic. The first reason is that drugs and alcohol may contribute to the development of schizophrenia or precipitate its expression in already vulnerable individuals. This in turn would enhance co-morbidity rates. Second, it can be due to enhanced awareness of the problem among clinicians.

Third, the harmful effects of prolonged drug addiction to the central nervous system including brain damage can lead to substance-induced psychosis. However, the occurrence of psychosis may be together or long after the cessation of drug addiction. Rounsaville (2007) described this in details:

> If psychotic symptoms emerge during periods of heavy drug use, these may indeed be "substance induced," but they may also be manifestations of an independent illness that happens to be emerging at the same time or that may be precipitated by the concurrent substance use. (Rounsaville, 2007:948)

Rounsaville (2007) further articulated that there is usually a period of being drug-free before the concurrence of drug addiction and schizophrenia. It may occur in adolescence or early adulthood. The sustained drug-free period may be long enough to question whether or not the onset of schizophrenia is drug induced or merely caused by other related psychosocial factors.

It is difficult to establish or practice precise guidelines for specifying the amount of time that defines a "sustained drug-free period."

Prevalence of Substance Abused Psychosis

Rounsaville (2007), according to related studies, concluded that in patients with stimulant-induced psychoses, 1%–15% had psychotic symptoms that persisted greater than one month. Further complications arise for patients who abuse multiple substances, each of which with a differing profile of psychotogenic effects and duration of withdrawal syndromes. Also, patients with co-morbid psychotic disorders and substance abuse are likely to have a poor memory of the precise sequence of events that occurred during their teens, such as pinpointing the onset of initial psychotic symptoms versus the initiation of heavy substance use.

A recent review of stimulant-induced psychosis documented the following rates of reported symptoms: paranoia (25%–75%), auditory hallucinations (50%–80%), ideas of references (15%–60%), Schneiderian first-rank symptoms (up to 50%), and negative symptoms (5%–30%).

INTERPRETATION OF DRUG ADDICTION AND SCHIZOPHRENIA

Complexity of Concurrence of Drug Addiction and Schizophrenia

Prolonged drug addiction has a high co-morbidity with schizophrenia. Conceptually, there may be three different types of positions regarding the relationship between schizophrenia and drug addiction. They are listed as follows:

1) Prolonged drug addiction leads to schizophrenia
2) Schizophrenia is coped with and delayed by spontaneous drug addiction
3) Drug addiction goes with schizophrenia

Prolonged Drug Addiction Leads to Schizophrenia

Regarding position 1, drug addiction leads to various types of mental illnesses, there can be three different types of causes.

1A. Prolonged drug addiction creates irreversible harm to the central nervous system, which leads to mental confusion and occurrence of schizophrenia.
1B. Prolonged drug addiction nurtures drug-related interpersonal and psychosocial traumas that leads to occurrence of schizophrenia.

1C. Prolonged drug addiction creates irreversible harm to organs such as the liver, bladder, and kidneys. Deterioration and failure of organs nurture mental stress to the individual with a result of schizophrenia.

In position 1, 1A and 1B mostly commonly occur in clients with prolonged drug addiction. In position 1A, it has long been biochemically proven that prolonged intake of substances, in particular amphetamines, should have an adverse effect on the central nervous system, which can lead to schizophrenia.

Also, prolonged intake of methamphetamines will possibly alter the activity of the dopamine system that can lead to recurrence of psychotic symptoms.

For position 1B, prolonged drug addiction nurtures drug-related interpersonal and psychosocial traumas that leads to occurrence of schizophrenia. The following description can describe this in detail:

> As the night wore on, he explained to me that when he smoked crystal meth, he could sit for hours on end with his eyes shut, imagining himself climbing mountains and surviving snow avalanches, or going on heroic journeys through deep tropical jungles.
>
> "Once, I sat there for three straight days and explored these caves until I found the ruins of an ancient underground kingdom with huge castles and pyramids. When Crystal ran out of her love, I went and got more so I could continue with the adventure."
>
> This would often continue for up to 18 hours at a time. After years of going on these adventures, Bernard woke up to find he no longer had his job, or his salary, or his house—all of which, in turn, led him to smoke more meth. (Williams 2007:35)

That means, there is a vicious cycle in which the more the client engages and absorbs in amphetamine addiction, the more s/he is socially excluded and isolated. Finally, s/he may lose his/her job, salary, house, family, and respect from others.

All these show that the prolonged stimulating effects of these drugs may contribute to the onset of schizophrenia. First, in taking amphetamines, individuals feel highly excited and agitated. In doing so, both their physical and mental activities are highly stimulated. Together with these can be the occurrence of flight of ideas such as grandiose delusions and hallucinations. Some individuals may delude that they are superman/woman that can fly out their window. Some may even think that they become cleverer than before with lot of ideas to win horseracing and lotteries. Some become very brave and courageous to perform those duties and activities that they rarely dare to do so in normal times. A timid man who wants to but dare not chase beautiful girls may suddenly become very open and aggressive in initiate courtship. Gradually, individuals are not addicted to taking amphetamines but rather they are addicted to drug-induced grandiose delusions. As their addiction increases, so does the grandiosity of their drug-induced hallucinations and delusions. It becomes more and more similar to grandiose delusions in schizophrenia. After several years of chronic, heavy, and severe addiction of amphetamines, the occurrence of grandiose delusions occurs automatically even without drug taking.

A similar situation happens in taking hallucinogens in which favorable visual or auditory hallucinations are induced by the effect of hallucinogens. Individuals addicted to hallucinogens often proclaim that all these drug-induced hallucinations are highly stimulating and gratifying their unfulfilled wishes. A student who looks for good grades in a coming tough examination, after taking marijuana (a kind of hallucinogen), may say that s/he deludes that s/he has already gotten and is enjoying the very good grade in this examination. All these drug-induced hallucinations are very attractive and seductive to related individuals making them more and more absorbed in that, and they finally become addicted to hallucinogens. As s/he becomes a chronic user, related hallucinations are highly intensified and fragmented.

Finally, even all these hallucinations occur spontaneously even without drug taking. At that moment, hallucinogen-induced psychosis should be formed. Together with drug-induced traumas, the content of hallucinations may change accordingly from unfulfilled wishes to related traumatic memories.

However, the tranquilizing effects of the drug also hinder his/her overall ego and social functioning, making the individual become more and more inert, passive, and withdrawn. That means, their repression mechanism of traumatic memories and experiences increases because of the tranquilizing effects of related drugs. As the addiction of tranquilizers increases, the individual may finally become highly inert, passive, and withdrawn from reality. That mean, s/he may be deeply regressive and unable to perform normal roles in family, work, and normal social interaction. As social isolation and self-isolation increase, the individual may finally suffer from self-breaking and the onset of schizophrenia. However, the onset does not start with active positive symptoms of schizophrenia, such as prevailing paranoid and/or grandiose delusions and hallucinations. Instead, it may manifest in a form of negative symptoms such as alogia (difficulties in speech and expression), anhedonia (difficulties in social interaction and search for happiness), avolition (difficulties in meaningful actions and behaviors), and blunted affect (difficulties in having normal affective responses). That means, traumatic repression with numbing of senses and responses finally turn into intensive regression in which alogia can be regarded as extreme repression of speech and expression; anhedonia can be regarded as extreme repression of social interaction and search for happiness; avolition can be regarded as extreme repression of meaningful actions and behaviors; and blunt affect can be regarded as extreme repression of normal affective responses.

In position 1C, ketamines are a good example in which prolonged addiction leads to toxification of the body, including the following:

- Cardiovascular: abnormal heart rhythms, slow heart rate or fast heart rate, high blood pressure or low blood pressure
- Central nervous system: Ketamine is traditionally avoided in people with or at risk of intracranial hypertension (ICP) due to concerns about ketamine causing increased intracranial pressure. It does not increase ICP more than opioids.[58]
- Dermatologic: Transient reddening of the skin, transient measles-like rash

- Gastrointestinal: reduced appetite, nausea, increased salivation, vomiting
- Local: Pain, eruptions or rashes at the injection site
- Neuromuscular and skeletal: Increased skeletal muscle tone (tonic-clonic movements)
- Ocular: Double vision, increased intraocular pressure, involuntary eye movements, tunnel vision
- Respiratory: Airway obstruction, cessation of breathing, increased bronchial secretions, reduced effort to breathe, spasm of the vocal cords (larynx)
- Other: Anaphylaxis, dependence, emergence reaction (Lexi 2014: 6)

Apart from all these bodily symptoms, there are also urinary tract symptoms that cause a permanent harmful effect on the bladder.

> Urinary tract symptoms have been collectively referred as "ketamine-induced ulcerative cystitis" or "ketamine-induced vesicopathy," and they include urge *incontinence*, decreased *bladder* compliance, decreased bladder volume, *detrusor* overactivity, and painful *blood in urine*. *Bilateral hydronephrosis* and *renal papillary necrosis* have also been reported in some cases. (Lexi 2014:9)

Coupled with permanent damage on the central nervous system and the out-of-body experiences, many prolonged users of ketamine may develop schizophrenia. The following narration from a client with prolonged ketamine abuse and psychosis may illustrate this briefly. Related parties' consensus to use their stories for academic purposes was sought. For the sake of confidentiality, personal identities and information are properly disguised.

> Kerry: I took ketamine when I was sixteen years ago. I came from a broken family in which my mother ran away when I was only five years. My father got another woman who did not care for me. I was frequently

bullied by schoolmates. I was depressed, confused, and frustrated in my childhood and adolescence.

One of my classmates persuaded me to take ketamine at a party. From that time onward, I was addicted to ketamine. It really helped me to get rid of life's frustration and unhappiness. I worked part-time to earn money to buy ketamine. I was so fond of the k-hole experience. It gave me a sense of being disconnected from my body. It separated me from frustrated reality. It was a type of comatose-like state. I felt flying in the universe. The more frustrated in daily life, the more I got into ketamine addiction.

When I graduated from secondary school, I had already become a chronic ketamine user. I found a full-time job doing manual labor for moving company. At first, everything seemed all right. I worked in the daytime and took ketamine at night. Gradually, the prolonged harmful effect of ketamine began to swallow my life. Even in the daytime, I was a bit confused in driving. I always harbored uncontrollable flashbacks in my brain. It caused a serious accident. Fortunately, no one was hurt in the accident. I lost my job. I took another one as a worker in a fast food shop where I had to be highly efficient in facing a lot of customers. At that moment, my urinary tract symptoms appeared. My bladder was hurt in prolonged ketamine toxic damage. I needed to go to toilet every twenty minutes. Because of that I was unemployed. My parents knew that I was addicted to ketamine.

After a serious quarrel and fight with my father, I left my parents' house. I was homeless, unemployed, and addicted to ketamine. I slept on the street at night, and during the day, I tried to find some casual job to survive. However, my ketamine addiction urinary tract symptoms made me jobless, and I became a beggar, begging for money. I was poor, helpless, and worthlessness. occasionally, I stole and picked pockets.

One day, I was too weak and fainted in the street. Someone called the police and I was sent to the hospital. The psychiatrist there diagnosed me as suffering from ketamine addiction and paranoid schizophrenia. Regarding the urinary tract symptoms, the medical practitioner said my bladder was seriously hurt by prolonged ketamine addiction. An operation was done to improve the function of the bladder. Two months later, I was discharged from the hospital and sent to a detoxification center. Frankly speaking, when my health condition improved and I regained the dignity of being a person, my paranoid delusions were lessened.

Schizophrenia Is Coped with and Delayed by Spontaneous Drug Addiction

Regarding position 2, onset of schizophrenia is delayed and coped with by drug addiction. It can be done in several ways.

2A. Drug addiction enables the individual to escape from the painfully oppressive reality thus delayed psychotic nurtures by oppressive reality.
2B. Drug addiction provides the individual a means to suppress and repress the recall and rebound of various kinds of traumas that provoke the onset of schizophrenia.
2C. Drug addiction alters the state of mind and body of the individual. At the same time, it also alters the individual's psychosocial and physical condition that leads to schizophrenia.

These three positions coincided with the Smith and Hucker (1995) comprehensive review of related studies on reasons for substance abuse by people with schizophrenia. First, those clients with better premorbid adjustment are more sociable and therefore exposed to more opportunities to experiment with illicit drugs and alcohol. Second, after the onset of the schizophrenic psychosis, clients use drugs to cope with stress related to psychotic symptoms.

Third, in some subcultures, the label of drug addict is more acceptable than a psychotic patient. Fourth, the effect of substance abuse can mediate symptoms of schizophrenia. Psychostimulant drugs may reduce negative symptoms, such as apathy and withdrawal, whereas alcohol and benzodiazepines can temporarily suppress psychotic symptoms; a possibility is that psychostimulant drugs counteract distressing neuroleptic-induced extrapyramidal side effects, particularly akathisia. Hallucinogens and amphetamines may, at the same time, deter the onset of psychosis. For those clients with intensive traumas in their childhood and adolescence, they may need intensive psychic and mental energy to repress the triggering and rebound of these traumatic experiences and memories. Otherwise, frequent rebound and triggering of trauma may result in intensive self-breaking. As a consequence, they are vulnerable to self-fragmentation and the onset of schizophrenia.

To reactivate related internal psychic and mental energy, these clients may incline to take hallucinogens and amphetamines. Under those sorts of conditions, drug-induced hallucinations may be highly various among individuals. Some may have grandiose hallucinations with contents of unfulfilled wishes (Type 1). Some may have triggering of previous traumatic memories (Type 2). Some may have a mixture of both (Type 3). In normal cases, individuals may first have Type 1 hallucinations and feel happy about that.

Their mental and psychic energy is activated by the delusive actualization of their unfulfilled wishes induced by the drug effects. Under that sort of condition, the onset of psychosis may thus be deterred. Later, as the drug addiction grows and persists, mental and psychic energy activated by drugs exhaust the individual's residual ego strengths and energy. Consequently, individual's residual energy to suppress his/her traumatic memories is exhausted. Thus, drug-induced hallucination tends to be Type 2, triggering of previous traumatic memories. The rebound of these traumatic memories gradually intensifies in forms of paranoid delusions and hallucinations.

At that moment, it is actually the onset of schizophrenia. If the client is continuously addicted to amphetamines and hallucinogens, the content of the hallucinations may finally be a combination of both Type 1 and Type 2 together. Unfulfilled wishes in Type 1 hallucinations may finally intensify to form grandiose hallucinations. In severe cases, individuals may even change their self-identities to delusive grandiose identities. A combination of Type 1 and Type 2 may finally become a shift between paranoid and grandiose delusions and hallucinations.

The situation may be different if the individual is addicted to tranquilizers. The effects of tranquilizers make them feel calm, peaceful, and in many ways detached from painful, abusive, and oppressive reality in their family, community, and society. By doing so, it can deter or delay the onset of schizophrenia.

Drug Addiction Goes with Schizophrenia

Regarding position 3, drug addiction goes with schizophrenia. It can also happen in several ways:

3A. Schizophrenia occurs before the intake of drugs (mixing with the withdrawal effects of drugs)
3B. Schizophrenia occurs during the intake of drugs (co-morbid with the stimulating effects of drugs)
3B. Schizophrenia occurs immediately after the intake the drugs (co-morbid after the diminishing stimulating effects of drugs)
3D. Schizophrenia occurs long after the intake of drugs

These four positions can be elaborated in terms of altered states of consciousness. In fact, both the drug-stimulated episode and psychotic symptoms are altered states of consciousness.

Ludwig defined the altered state of consciousness as follows:

> An altered state is any mental state(s), induced by various physiological, psychological, or pharmacological maneuvers or agents, which can be recognized subjectively by the individual himself (or by an objective observer of the individual) as representing a sufficient deviation in subjective experience of psychological functioning from certain general norms for that individual during alert, waking consciousness (Ludwig 1966:225).

Tart (1969) defined it as the subjective experience of a state of consciousness and its deviation from a normal waking state. Vaitl (2012) distinguished the altered state of consciousness in terms of:

- Spontaneous (daydreaming and near-death experience)
- Physical and physiological (fasting and sex)
- Psychological (music, meditation, hypnosis)
- Pathological (epilepsy, brain damage)

- Pharmacological (psychoactive substances)

Vaitl (2012) further suggests four basic aspects of experiences in altered states of consciousness:

1) activation
2) awareness span
3) self-awareness
4) sensory dynamics

Dittrich (1998) suggested three basic dimensions in altered states of consciousness:

1) oceanic boundlessness
2) dread of ego dissolution
3) visionary restructuralization

Oceanic boundlessness (OB) measures derealization and depersonalization phenomena associated with a positive basic mood ranging from heightened feelings to sublime happiness or grandiosity. The second dimension, "dread of ego dissolution" (AED), measures thought disorder, ego disintegration, loss of autonomy, and self-control variously associated with arousal, anxiety, and paranoid feelings of being endangered. The third dimension, "visionary restructuralization" (VR), refers to auditory and visual illusions, hallucinations, synaesthesias, and changes in the meaning of various percepts.

Psychoactive drugs have a powerful effect on altered states of consciousness. Opiates include heroin and morphine and produces analgesia and feelings of euphoria. Opiates abuse the results in decreased production of endorphins in the brain. Cocaine alters one's state of consciousness, as it inhibits the reuptake of norepinephrine, serotonin, and dopamine. Lysergic acid diethylamide activates serotonin receptors. The abusers may alter quickly through a range from fear to ecstasy. Vollenweider and Geyer (2001) affirmed the altered state of consciousness in psychoactive drugs is, in many ways, similar to those in psychotic symptoms, in particular in AED and visual or auditory delusions. In other words, both psychotic experiences as drug-induced experiences are an altered state of consciousness in which the individual tries to escape from the painful reality. Gradually, even without the intake of psychoactive drugs, the individual may be self-absorbed in related altered states of consciousness. Gradually, altered states of consciousness can be self-induced even without the intake of psychoactive drugs.

TRAUMA AND SCHIZOPHRENIA

Yip (2014) has a comprehensive review on trauma and schizophrenia. Prolonged and severe trauma, in particular childhood abuse, can contribute to the development of schizophrenia. Clinically, it is a severe dissociation effect after post-traumatic fear that gradually develops into self-fragmentation in schizophrenia.

From Traumatic Dissociation to Schizophrenic Self-Fragmentation

Breaking Down of the Ego System in Post-Trauma Fear

Garland (1998) affirmed trauma is a strong breaking effect on individual's ego system

> The individual, without an integrated and cohesive ego system, in facing the traumatic event, is unable to deal with the adverse stimuli constructively. S/he is lack of an internal apparatus to contain, to interpret, and to incorporate all these negative stimuli into the ego system. Instead, the overwhelming negative stimuli may be intensive and strong enough to break the already fragile and loose ego system. The impacts of powerful negative stimuli from traumatic events stir up the early phantasies of devastation and cruelty of the individual. (Garland 1998: 45)

The longer traumatic experiences are, the greater and longer the emotional loading to the individual and the more vulnerable s/he becomes in facing both external and internal adverse demands and stimuli. Very often, it is not the actual traumatic experiences that matter. Instead, it is how the individual contains, selects, interprets, recalls, and filters the traumatic experiences. The breaking down of the individual's ego system in traumatic events is based on four groups of related factors (Yip 2014).

Group A: Destructive effects of the traumatic experiences (intensity, duration, and frequency of harm created)

Group B: Durability of the ego system in facing external threat (stability and integrity of the ego system, as well as unsettled and unresolved emotional complex)

Group C: Related support from external environment (support, care, comfort, and acceptance from others. Or rejection, isolation, stigmatization, exclusion, and punishment from others)

Group D: Inner processing of traumatic experience (filtering, containing, interpreting, repressing, and recalling of traumatic experiences

Following Freud's line of thinking, Garland (1998) described the breaking down process after traumatic experiences in detail.

Garland (1998) described that there is a breakdown of one's normal ego functioning and defense mechanism in life in facing traumatic experiences. Yip (2013) concluded that the breakdown of the ego system includes the following:

1) a breakdown of an established way of going about one's life
2) a breakdown of established beliefs
3) a breakdown about the predictability of established mental structures
4) a breakdown of established defensive organization
5) a breakdown of the trust in the fundamental goodness of one's objects

6) a breakdown of protective function of the good objects
7) a breakdown of the world itself
   (Garland 1998: 10)

Following this initial breakdown is a chronic fear and paranoid belief about one's status in the world. That means the individual's senses of substantiality, cohesiveness, and integrity are gradually shattered. Externally, s/he becomes oversensitive and overresponsive to external threats and difficulties. Internally, s/he loses his/her defense, competence, beliefs, trust, and predictability in facing frustration in reality. In other words, apart from the fear of breakdown, the individual's fear is generally transformed into a primitive paranoia toward the external world as well as his/her ability and life. Within Garland's formulation, the ego system is not only breaking but can split into various parts. The individual's ego takes a part of it and transfers this part into the lost objects. The transformation is completed by a full identification of the lost objects. According to Yip (2013), within this transformation, the individual actually undergoes several inner psychic processes as the following:

1) splitting the ego into at least two parts (one part represents the ego itself, one part represents the lost object. In some case, according to Klein, the splitting can be further. The part representing the ego itself can further split into good and bad self. The part representing the lost object can further split into good and bad other)
2) strong and unconscious identification with the lost object
3) fantasy that the part of ego has actually become the lost object

This is a complicated process. The individual avoids the fear of breaking of the ego system by sealing up this fear through dissociation of mind, body, and external perception. Then, the individual tries to deny related loss in the trauma by splitting part of the ego and identifying with the lost object. These three mechanisms are closely related to one another. It is a combination of three crucial mental processes that occur in schizophrenia, depression, and trauma.

1) Self-splitting in the schizoid self-fragmentation (schizophrenia)
2) Identification of lost object in the depressive self-introjection (depression)
3) Dissociation of body, mind, or memory in the traumatic experience and recall (trauma)

However, all these mental processes are only in an initial stage. The self-splitting process only occurs in a slight way. The splitting process stops when the split ego part can identify the lost object by introjecting the symbols of the lost object. The self-splitting will not go further to a stage of self-fragmentation as in people with schizophrenia. The identification and introjection of the lost object only occurs in an initial stage. As far as the lost object is symbolized and introjected by the split part of ego, the process of introjection stops. It will not go further to a stage of severe depression with intense guilt and worthlessness. The dissociation of body, mind, or memory also occurs, but it stops as the lost objects is symbolized and introjected by the split part of the ego. The individual does not need not to further the dissociation process with severe malfunctioning of bodily and ego functioning (Yip 2013). In other words, these three mechanisms interact and counteract with one another. In other words, if the individual can use these three mechanisms together, s/he is able to avoid being fixated in any one of them. If either the dissociation mechanism or the introjection mechanism fails, the individual has to involve fully in the self-breaking mechanism that may finally lead to the onset of schizophrenia.

Trauma, Abuse, Victimization, and Psychosis

In recent years, there is plenty of research evidence showing that psychosis is closely related to trauma (Larkin and Morrison 2006) in the following ways:

a) Child abuse, victimization, and psychosis
b) PTSD in response to acute psychosis

c) Psychosis with co-morbidity of PTSD
d) Internal process from traumatic memories, emotions, and negative self to psychosis

In this section, the writer is going to describe every one of them in detail:

Child Abuse, Victimization, and Psychosis

The study by Holowka et al. (2003) showed that among adult outpatients with schizophrenia, 35% of them suffered from emotional abuse, 42% with physical neglect, and 73% of them had emotional neglect by their parents during their childhood. Many studies showed that there was a high correlation between child abuse and hallucination. Read and Argyle (1999) showed that for those subjects with former child sex abuse experiences, 53% of them demonstrated some forms of hallucination. For those with physical abuse experiences in childhood, 58% of them showed some forms of auditory hallucinations. For subjects with both types of experiences, 71% of them exhibited auditory hallucinations. Also, hallucinations are particularly common in incest survivors (Ellenson 1985; Read and Argyle 1999).

Regarding the content of hallucinations, many studies showed that clients with sexual abuse or physical abuse history in childhood may harbor hallucinations with refined details of such experiences. In some cases, clients may even harbor a highly symbolized delusive hallucination (Famularo et al. 1992).

Trauma and Psychosis: Co-morbidity

Strauss et al. (2011) had reviewed related studies and concluded that co-morbidity between PTSD and schizophrenia is around 19% to 66%. Based on this review, they described that positive, negative, and first-rank symptoms in schizophrenia are all influenced by the occurrence of PTSD.

Psychotic positive symptoms for people with co-morbid PTSD and schizophrenia have more frequent violent thoughts, behaviors, and feelings, as well as heightened paranoia, greater severity of delusion, and hallucinations.

Regarding psychotic first-rank symptoms, people with co-morbid schizophrenia and PTSD had more negative beliefs about self and others that may mediate the relationship between trauma and paranoia. Also their reexperiencing symptoms may mediate the link between trauma and paranoid hallucination.

For psychotic negative symptoms, the presence of PTSD in schizophrenia was associated with an increase in secondary negative symptoms.

Internal Process from Trauma to Psychosis

There is a growing literature showing that psychosis is a prolonged result of PTSD. Jankowski et al. (2006) summed up the process from PTSD to psychosis in the following way:

> The basic thesis is that the psychosis itself, characterized by perceptual disturbances, frightening delusions, feelings of persecution, and other threats to the self, may be sufficiently terrifying to qualify as "traumatic events" according to criterion A of DSM IV. This concept represents a modification of the traditional PTSD paradigm, which implies the traumatic stressor is an external event. (Jankowski et al. 2006: 88)

Regarding the process from PTSD to psychosis, there are a number of studies describing the details. Most of them are within a cognitive behavioral orientation. Fowler et al. (2006) tried to speculate the pathway from trauma to psychosis within four cognitive routes:

1) Direct associations between intrusive memories of traumatic or stressful experiences and delusion and hallucination.
2) Indirect association between trauma and persecutory delusions and hallucinations mediated by negative evaluation of self and others (the schema route).
3) Indirect association between trauma and hallucination mediated by negative and self-critical rumination of relationship between the voices hearer and the voice identity.
4) Speculations about potential catastrophic interactions between trauma processes and information processing abnormalities which characterize psychosis which may magnify vulnerability to psychosis. (Fowler et al. 2006: 100)

Direct Associations between Intrusive Memories and Persecutory Hallucinations

The first cognitive route is the direct association between intrusive memories of traumatic experiences and delusions and hallucinations. There is consistent evidence that a traumatic history can increase the risk of psychosis.

The severity of hallucination is associated with the degree of hurt and harm in sex abuse (Bebbington et al. 2004; Fowler et al. 2006). Morrison (2001) affirmed that normal intrusive memories in forms of image and voices in the state of anxiety and other neurotic disorders can be gradually transformed into delusion and hallucination. The study by Fowler (1997) showed that there were four cases with a direct connection between traumatic events, such as being raped and being bullied, and experiences of hallucinations. In these four cases, clients all harbored related auditory hallucinations in forms of critical comments and threatening from the abusers.

Indirect Association between Trauma and Persecutory Hallucination with Negative View on Self and Others

Regarding indirect linkage between trauma and persecutory delusions and hallucinations, related studies showed that it is mediated by negative evaluation of self and others within a schema route. Recent studies (Fowler et al. 1997) showed that persecutory ideas and hallucinations are related to a negative view of self and related negative emotions. It appears in a form of a vicious cycle. The more negative one's self esteem and emotions is, the more one becomes vulnerable to external negative comment. Then, all these negative emotions and self-appreciation gradually turn into persecutory hallucinations. The combination of anxiety and negative self-evaluation may directly relate to positive psychotic experiences (Fowler et al. 2006: 110). Persecutory hallucinations and delusions can also relate to negative views of others in which individuals assume that others have imposed harm, hurt, oppression, and criticism on them. (Fowler et al. 2006).

In many ways, the negative views of self and others can come together within the experiences and recall of traumatic experiences. Fowler et al. (2006) believed that the occurrence of persecutory delusions and hallucinations are not only a defensive response to negative self-esteem (Bentall et al. 2001) but a catastrophic appraisal of social position of an extreme negative self and negative others. The Fowler et al. (2006) study concluded the following:

> The combined pattern of extreme self and other evaluation was associated with a history of humiliating trauma (bullying, assault, sexual abuse) and multiple regressions suggested that extreme self and other evaluations were the strongest mediator of the relationship between traumatic events and paranoia….We have found clear evidence to suggest that extreme negative evaluation of self and others are more likely to be present among people with psychosis who have been exposed to either ongoing social adversity or specific social humiliation such as rape or bullying. The way in which past traumatic and stressful experiences may be linked to paranoia may then be via the mediating or negative self and others evaluations. This can occur as a result of adaptation and social learning in a similar manner to that suggested by psychological theorists of PTSD. (Fowler et al. 2006: 111)

Traumatic experiences and recall are correlated with negative evaluation of self and others as well as negative emotions, such as anger, depression, and feelings of being threatened.

Indirect Association between Trauma and Hallucination Mediated by Negative and Self-Critical Rumination of Relationships between the Voices Hearer and the Voice Identity

Many studies showed that hallucinations can be regarded as misattribution of one's own thoughts or internal dialogue because of self-monitoring and faulty interpretation of external stimuli (Bentall 1990) There is also evidence that auditory hallucination is a sign of being humiliated and oppressed in the external environment. The voice heard is closely related to the dominating and powerful persecutors within all these humiliating experiences.

Speculations about Potential Catastrophic Interactions between Trauma Processes and Information Processing Abnormalities, Which Characterize Psychosis, Which May Magnify Vulnerability to Psychosis

In this cognitive route, severe negative views of self and others may finally distort the individual's normal information processing. Cognitions with internal origins, such as images and thought, are regarded as external origins in terms of hallucinations and delusions (Hemsely 1994). Individuals' negative views of self and others are further provoked and nurtured by spontaneous fear and continuous occurrence and recall of traumatic experiences. Under that condition, their cognitive process is greatly distorted. They have impairment in inputting new and spontaneous information from external reality. Instead, their cognitive processing is greatly distorted by prevailing negative emotions and recall of memories of traumatic experiences.

TRAUMA, SCHIZOPHRENIA, AND DRUG ADDICTION: IMPLICATIONS TO PSYCHOSOCIAL INTERVENTION

As mentioned in previous chapter, there are four routes and combinations of trauma, mental illness, and drug addiction. They are listed as follows:

1) T leads to M, D is used to cope with M and T (trauma leads to psychosis. Drug addiction is used to cope with trauma and psychosis).
2) D is used to cope with T. Prolonged D leads to Td and related Md (Drug addiction is used to cope with trauma. Prolonged drug addiction leads to drug-led trauma and drug-induced psychosis).
3) D is used to cope with M. Prolonged D leads to Td and related Md (Drug addiction is used to cope with psychosis. Prolonged drug addiction leads to drug-led trauma and drug-induced psychosis).
4) D leads to Md and Td, further intensive D to cope with Md and Td (Drug addiction leads to drug-induced psychosis and drug-led trauma. Further intensive drug addiction to cope with drug-induced psychosis and drug-led trauma).

Most of four positions have been covered in previous discussions in trauma and schizophrenia, as well as the complexity of psychosis and drug addiction. The most important clarification is three different type of traumas:

1) Trauma may not lead to psychosis (T1)
2) Trauma that leads to psychosis (T2)
3) Trauma induced by prolonged drug addiction in particular in chronic drug addiction (T3)

Similarly, there are three types of psychosis:

1) Psychosis occurred before drug addiction (P1)
2) Psychosis induced by drug addiction biochemically (P2)
3) Psychosis induced by drug addiction psychosocially (P3)
4) Psychosis goes together with drug addiction (P4)

All these have very important implications to related psychosocial intervention to clients with drug addictions.

In Route 1: Trauma Leads to Psychosis. Drug Addiction Is Used to Cope with Trauma and Psychosis

In this route, trauma leads to psychosis. That means, trauma is (T2). Also, psychosis occurs before drug addiction (P1). That means, psychosocial intervention should be focused on resolving traumas. Clients may suffer from child abuse. Related traumas embrace strong breaking effects and induced splitting effects of the ego system. The individual is accustomed to using drug addiction to cope with the breaking effects of the trauma. In other words, psychosocial intervention to the client in this route should be focused on:

1) Accept and understand clients using drug addiction to cope with related traumas, in particular those in childhood.
2) Avoid persuading or deterring clients to engage in drug addiction.
3) Facilitate clients to share their previous traumatic experiences in a natural, non-harmful way.
4) Enable clients to resolve clients' traumatic experience and memories appropriately.
5) Develop clients' constructive and positive daily habit and hobbies to cope with stress related to past traumatic memories.

When these five intervention procedures can be attained, the clients are ready to be rid of their drug addiction.

In Route 2: Drug Addiction Is Used to Cope with Trauma. Prolonged Drug Addiction Leads to Drug-Led Trauma and Drug-Induced Psychosis

In this route, trauma is not inducing psychosis (T1). However, the individual is accustomed to using drug addiction to cope with life stress and unpleasant memories. There may be several reasons behind this pathological coping mechanism. First, individuals may have a thin social support system in which they are unable to get any support from others. Second, individuals may face a highly oppressive social environment in which they can only suppress their inner pain and traumatic memory experiences by regular and prolonged addiction.

Third, previous trauma may be highly insidious and shameful, such as sex abuse, domestic violence, and parental oppression that cannot be shared or voiced out by others. Drug addiction is certainly a fixated, unchangeable coping to life stress and hardship.

Psychosis is drug induced (P2). That means, in the treatment and recovery process, the first priority should be to focus on establishing a good support system so that clients can seek help, support, and ventilate related stress, negative emotions, and hardships from significant others rather than fixation on drug addiction. Thus, related psychosocial intervention in this route should be:

1) A full understanding of clients' social support system; see whether they have enough social support or their significant others are supportive, oppressive, or abusive.
2) It is important to facilitate clients to establish a good social support system with good significant others.
3) Enable clients to share and voice out their negative emotions, stress, hardships, and unpleasant memories with good significant others.
4) Help clients to develop good habits such as physical exercises and healthy hobbies so that they can regularize their negative emotions, stress, hardships, and unpleasant memories daily without depending on drug addiction.
5) Enable clients to rehabilitate and recover from drug addiction.
6) Related treatment to drug-induced psychosis. Very often when drug addiction is in recovery, drug-induced psychosis diminishes accordingly.
7) Deep healing of related trauma, in particular those insidious and shameful ones.

In Route 3: Drug Addiction Is Used to Cope with Psychosis. Prolonged Drug Addiction Leads to Drug-Led Trauma and Drug-Induced Psychosis

In this route, psychosis (P1) occurs before drug addiction. It may not relate to explicit childhood trauma such as abuse, nor it is related to severe incidental traumas. It can originate from a highly engulfing psychosocial development in childhood and adolescence. Drug addiction is used to enable the individual to escape from an engulfing social environment. Gradually, the individual is accustomed to drug addiction as a fixated way to escape from an unpleasant and engulfing environment. However, prolonged and chronic addiction leads to drug-led traumas (T3), such as financial difficulties, social exclusion, and self-isolation, with a result of psychosis (P2). Drug-induced psychosis (P3) is because of biochemical harm on the central nervous system by the toxic effects of prolonged addiction. In this route, schizophrenic conditions are highly complicated. Clients can suffer from three types of psychoses. Unlike route 2, there is only drug-induced psychosis. Once drug addiction ceases, the psychotic condition can be enlightened or even diminished. In this route, P1 and P2 reinforces one another. Schizophrenic conditions are chronic and have long been precipitated by an engulfing social environment, social exclusion, and self-isolation. Related hallucinations and delusions can be highly stable, organized, and penetrating in most aspects of life. In this prolonged and chronic psychotic condition, coupled with a decrease of social functioning because of chronic drug addiction and habitual escape and detachment from reality, clients can first have prevailing positive and first-rank symptoms but subsided by drug addiction. In the P2 and P3 condition, negative symptoms can be dominating.

They may need prolonged dependence on related psychiatric rehabilitation. Thus, psychosocial intervention in the process of recovery in this route should be focused on the complexity of psychosis in different stages of drug addiction. Related psychosocial intervention can be listed out as follows:

1) A full understanding of various forms (P1, P2, and P3) of psychoses in the drug addiction, including forms, details, process, and contents of related symptoms.
2) Related symptoms in P1, P2, and P3 should be related to suffering, hardship, and stress in the psychosocial environment in clients' different life stages.
3) For P2 with prevailing positive symptoms P3 with prevailing negative symptoms, clients are accustomed to detach and isolate from reality. Thus, it is important that related professionals can help clients to improve their engagement in reality, including normal daily activities within the community and neighborhood, normal social interaction with significant others, normal daily rhythm, normal interest, hobbies, and engagement. Only by doing so, clients' social functioning can be enhanced and related positive and negative symptoms can be alleviated.
4) Psychosocial interventions on P1, P2, and P3 should be accompanied by appropriate medication, accommodation, vocational rehabilitation, financial aid, and social and recreational services in psychiatric rehabilitation.
5) When P1, P2, and P3 are gradually under control, drug addiction detoxification, rehabilitation can be rendered.

In Route 4: Drug Addiction Leads to Drug-Induced Psychosis and Drug-Led Trauma. Further Intensive Drug Addiction to Cope with Drug-Induced Psychosis and Drug-Led Trauma

In this route, drug addiction is one of the most crucial factors leading to drug-induced psychosis (P2: drug-induced psychosis biochemically and drug-led trauma [T3]). In many cases, clients reach a rock bottom stage in which there may be three possible outcomes. The first is overdose leading to sudden accidental death. The second is the accumulated pain and plight to an unbearable limit where clients may eventually commit suicide. The third is actively seeking or crying for help and becoming compliant clients in drug detoxification or psychiatric emergencies and rehabilitation services. Clients in this route may at first be highly resistant to formal service. They may harbor self-pride and narcissistic features on one hand, and with thin social support on the other hand. Even though related professionals actively approach them for service, they initially resist them. Not until they reach the rock bottom with severe chronic drug addiction, drug-led traumas, and drug-induced psychosis do they reconsider. Once they search for help from related professionals, it must be highly critical and urgent. Related professionals should be totally involved, genuine, and committed to helping clients in this rock bottom critical condition. Thus, related psychosocial intervention should be as follows:

1) Related professionals should be patient, genuine, and committed without being threatened by clients' high resistance in the service delivery. It is important, despite clients' resistance, related professionals should never terminate or close cases. They should maintain in regular contact with clients. Once clients' vicious cycle and rock bottom stage are reached, help must be rendered immediately.
2) When clients' critical conditions are discovered, related professionals should be fully committed and involved in crisis intervention, psychiatric emergencies to reduce possible risks of overdosage of drugs, suicidal attempts, and severe or critical medical conditions. Very often, immediate hospitalization and detoxification services are needed. In doing so, related professionals should be humanistic, genuine, and empathetic to clients' needs. Clients' dignity in the process of crisis intervention and psychiatric emergencies should be fully protected.
3) When harm reduction and detoxification is done, clients' drug addiction is alleviated and on the process of recovery. It is better for clients to stay in residential drug rehabilitation centers or drug detoxification centers for a long period of time, such as several months or one year, so that clients' vicious cycle of drug addiction, drug-induced psychosis, and drug-led traumas can be ceased by a

new rehabilitation life with new social network, new employment, and new accommodations.

4) When the rock bottom stage and critical condition are over and clients' drug addiction is detoxified, it is important for related professionals to establish trust and empathy with clients. Then under the help of professionals, clients should be facilitated to establish good social support systems and good hobbies to work out their frustrations in life.
5) At the same time, clients' drug-induced psychoses, drug-induced traumas, and drug-induced medical conditions should be much alleviated after a full and complete recovery from drug addiction. However, residual symptoms in drug-induced psychosis and drug-induced PTSD need to be addressed by appropriate psychosocial intervention and treatment.

Conclusion

This chapter is a comprehensive discussion about interpretation and intervention of drug addiction and psychosis. The chapter begins with a full articulation of etiology, diagnosis, and symptoms of schizophrenia. Diagnoses in DSM IV and DSM V are compared and discussed. Related literature review of co-morbidity of schizophrenia and drug addiction are thoroughly reviewed, including prevalence of schizophrenia and drug addiction, reasons why people with schizophrenia engage in substance abuse and drug addiction, as well as features and natures of drug-induced psychosis. Following this is a comprehensive interpretation of various positions in drug addiction and schizophrenia. It includes:

1) Prolonged drug addiction leads to schizophrenia.
2) Schizophrenia is coped with and delayed by spontaneous drug addiction.
3) Drug addiction goes with schizophrenia.

In each position, different types of manifestations are also discussed. The complexity of trauma, schizophrenia, and drug addiction are also comprehensively described. It starts with a theoretical underpinning of trauma and schizophrenia. Finally, different routes of traumas, schizophrenia, and drug addiction are reviewed. They are:

1) Trauma leads to psychosis. Drug addiction is used to cope with trauma and psychosis.
2) Drug addiction is used to cope with trauma. Prolonged drug addiction leads to drug-led trauma and drug-induced psychosis.
3) Drug addiction is used to cope with psychosis. Prolonged drug addiction leads to drug-led trauma and drug-induced psychosis.
4) Drug addiction leads to drug-induced psychosis and drug-led trauma. Further intensive drug addiction to cope with drug-induced psychosis and drug-led trauma.

Different routes imply different types of psychosis and traumas. It also implies a different focus on psychosocial intervention.

References

American Psychiatric Association (1994) *Diagnostic and Statistical Manual of Mental Disorder* (4th ed.) Washington, D.C: American Psychiatric Association.

American Psychiatric Association (2012) *Diagnostic and Statistical Manual of Mental Disorder* (5th ed.) Washington, D.C: American Psychiatric Association.

Andreasen N. C. (1984) *Scale for the Assessment of Negative Symptoms (SANS).* Iowa City, University of Iowa.

Bean. M. H. and Zinberg, N. E. (1981) (Edited) *Dynamic Approaches to the Understanding and Treatment of Alcoholism,* New York: Free Press.

Bebbington, P., Bhugra, D., Brugha, T., Singleton, N., Farrell, M., Jenkin, R. et al. (2004). Psychosis, victimization and childhood disadvantage: Evidence from the second British National Survey of Psychiatric Morbidity. *British Journal of Psychiatry*, 185: 220-226.

Bentall, R. P. (1990). The illusion of reality: A review and integration of psychological research on hallucination, *Psychological Bulletin*, 107: 82-85.

Bentall, R. P., Corcoran, R., Howard, R., Blackwood, R., and Kinderman, P. (2001). Persecutory delusions: A review and theoretical integration. *Clinical Psychology Review*, 21, 1143-1192.

Biskin, R. S. and Paris, J. (2013) Borderline personality disorder, alcohol use, bipolar disorder, comorbidity, *Psychiatry, Major Depressive Disorder, Mood Disorder and Personality Disorder,* 3(1): 440-62. https://www.borderline-personality-disorder.com/co-occuring-disorders/substance-abuse.

Blume, A. W. and Logan, D. (2013) Harm reduction approaches, *Interventions for Addiction*, 3: 633-642.

Bowen, M. (1976). Theory in the practice of psychotherapy. In Guerin, P. J. (Ed.), *Family therapy: Theory and practice* (pp. 42–90). New York: Gardner Press.

Bowen, M. (1978). *Family therapy in clinical practice.* New York: Jason Aronson.

Brennan, K. A., and Shaver, P. R. (1995). Dimensions of adult attachment, affect regulation, and romantic relationship functioning. *Personality and Social Psychology Bulletin,* 21, 267–283.

Briere, J. N. (1992) *Child Abuse Trauma: Theory and Treatment of the Lasting Effects*, London: Sage.

Carruth, B., and Burke, P. A. (2006) Psychological trauma and addiction treatment, B. Carruth Edited, *Psychological Trauma and Addiction Treatment*, New York: Haworth Press.

Caton, C. L. M., Drake, R. E., Hasin, R. S., Dominguez B., Shront D. E., Samet S., and Schanzer B. (2005) Difference between early phase primary psychotic disorder with concurrent substance use schizophrenia, *Archives of General Psychiatry*, 62: 137-143.

Cooper, M. L., Shaver, P. R., and Collins, N. L. (1998). Attachment styles, emotion regulation, and adjustment in adolescence. *Journal of Personality and Social Psychology*, 74, 1380–1397.

Descutner, C. J., and Thelen, M. H. (1991). Development and validation of a fear-of-intimacy scale. *Journal of Consulting and Clinical Psychology*, 3(2), 218–225.

Dittrich, A. (1998). The standardized psychometric assessment of altered state of consciousness, *Pharmacopsychiatry*, 3/Supple (S2): 80-4.

Dottan, R. F., Cohen, O., Iwaniec, D., Sapir, Y., and Weizman, A. (2003). The drug-user husband and his wife: Attachment styles, family cohesion and adaptability. *Journal of Substance Use and Misuse*, 38(2), 271–292.

Ellenson, G. (1985). Detecting a history of incest. *Social Casework*, November, 525-532.

Famularo, R., Kinscherff, R., and Fenton, T. (1992). Psychiatric diagnoses of maltreated children: Preliminary findings. *Journal of the American Academy of Children Adolescent Psychiatry,* 31, 863-867.

Fowler, D. (1997). Direct and indirect links between the content of psychotic symptoms and past traumatic experience: Evidence from therapists reports from the London-East Anlia study of cognitive behavior therapy for psychosis. *Paper presented at the British Association of Behavioral and Cognitive Psychotherapy Annual Conference*, Southport, Italy.

Fowler, D. Freeman, D., and Steel, C. et al. (2006). The catastrophic interaction hypothesis: How do stress, trauma, emotion In Larkin, W. and Morrison, A. P., (Edited) *Trauma and Psychosis: New Directions for Theory and Therapy. pp. 101-124.* London: Routledge.

Frankl, V. (1997). *Man's Search for Ultimate Meaning*. New York: Plenum.

Garland, C. (1998). 'Thinking about trauma' in C. Garland (Edited) *Understanding Trauma: A Psychoanalytical Approach*, pp.9-31. London: Duckworth.

Glasscote, R., Sussex, J. N., Jaffe, J. H., Ball, J., and Brill, J. (1972). *The Treatment of Drug Abuse: Programs, Problems, Prospects*. Washington, D. C.: Joint Information Service, APA and NIMH.

Hazan, C., and Shaver, P. (1987). Romantic love conceptualised as an attachment process. *Journal of Personality and Social Psychology*, 52: 511–524.

Hemsely, D. R. (1994). A cognitive model for schizophrenia and its neural basis, *Acta Psychiatric Scandinavia*, 90, 80-86.

Herman, J. (1992) *Trauma and Recovery*, New York: Basic Books.

Herman, J. L., Peery, C. and van der Kolk, B. A. (1989) Childhood trauma in borderline personality disorder, *American Journal of Psychiatry*, 146: 490-494.

Hoefler, D. Z., and Kooyman, M. (1996). Attachment transition, addiction and therapeutic bonding—An integrative approach. *Journal of Substance Abuse Treatment*, 13(6): 511–519.

Holowka, D., King, S., Saheb, D., Pukall, M., and Brunet, A. (2003). Childhood abuse and dissociative symptoms in adult schizophrenia. *Schizophrenia Research*, 60, 87-90.

Hong Kong government (2002) *A Report for the Tuen Mun Substance Abuse Outpatient Clinic*. Hong Kong Government.

Jankowski, M. K. Muser, K. T., and Rosenberg, S. D. (2006). Psychosis with comorbid PTSD, In Larkin, W. and Morrision, A. P., (Edited) *Trauma and Psychosis: New Directions for Theory and Therapy. pp. 75-100.* London: Routlege.

Jellinek, E. M. (1952) Phases of alcohol addition, *Quarterly Journal of Studies in Alcohol,* 13: 673-684.

Jellinek, E. M. (1960) *The Disease Concept of Alcoholism*, New Haven, Hillhouse Press.

Khantzian, E. J. (1980) An ego/self theory of substance dependence: A contemporary psychoanalytic perspective, *Theories of Drug Abuse: Selected Contemporary Perspective*, pp. 29-33. U.S.: National Institute on Drug Abuse.

Khantzian, E. J. (1981) Some treatment implication of the ego and self disturbances in alcoholism', In Bean. M. H. and Zinberg, N. E. (1981) (Edited) *Dynamic Approaches to the Understanding and Treatment of Alcoholism,* New York: Free Press.

Kilpatrick, D. G., Ruggiero, K. J., Acierno, R. Saunders, B. E., Resnick, H. S. and Best, C. L. (2003) Violence and risk of PTSD, major depression, substance abuse/dependence, and comorbity: Result from the national survey of adolescents, *Journal of Consulting and Clinical and Psychology*, 71(4): 692-700.

Larkin, W. and Morrision, A. P. (2006). (Edited) *Trauma and Psychosis: New Directions for Theory and Therapy*, London: Routlege.

Lexi, C. (2014) Merck manual; Drug information: Last full review/revision, *Ketamine Archived 9 March 2011 at the Wayback Machine.*

Links P. S., Steiner M. (1988) Psychopharmacologic management of patients with borderline personality disorder. *Canadian Journal of Psychiatry,* 33:355-359.

Liska, K. (1990) *Drug and the Human Body: With Implication for Society*, (4th Edition) New York; Macmillan Publishing Company.

Love and Respect Organization (2012) *What is Physical Abuse* http://www.loveisrespect.org/is-this-abuse/types-of-abuse/what-is-physical-abuse.

Ludwig, A. M. (1966) Altered states of consciousness, *Archives of General Psychiatry*, 15(3):225.

McGlashan, T. H. (1985) (Edited) *The Borderline: Current Empirical Research*, Washington, D.C.: American Psychiatric Association.

Miller, W. R. and Rollnick, S. (1991) *Motivational Intervention: Preparing People to Change Addictive Behaviors*, New York: The Guildford Press.

Morrison, S. P. (2001). The interpretation of intrusion in psychosis: An integrative cognitive approach to psychotic symptom, *Behavioral and Cognitive Psychotherapy*, 29, 257-276.

National Center on Child Abuse and Neglect (1988) N*ational Study of Incidence and Severity of Child Abuse and Neglect,* Washington, D.C. National Center on Child Abuse and Neglect.

National Institute of Drug Abuse (2013) *Long Term Effect of Methamphetamine* https://www.drugabuse.gov/publications/research-reports/methamphetamine/what-are-long-term-effects-methampheta mine-abuse.

National Society for Prevention of Cruelty to Children (NSPCC) (2010) *Child protection fact sheet The definitions and signs of child abuse,* NSPCC.

Peele, S. (1975) Love and Addiction, New York: Taplinger Publishing Company.

Peele, S. (1985) The Meaning of Addiction, Toronto: Lexington Books.

Prochasks, J. O., and Diclemente, C. C. (1982) *Trans-theoretical therapy: Towards a more integrative model of change; Psychotherapy, Theory, Research and Practice*, 19:276-288.

Read, J., and Argyle, N. (1999). Hallucination, delusions and thought disorders among adult psychiatric inpatients with a history of child abuse. *Psychiatric Services*, 50, 1467-1472.

Rollnick, S., Miller, W. R. and Butler, C. C. (2008) *Motivational Interviewing in Health Care*, New York: The Guildford Press.

Rounsaville, B. (2007) DSM V Research agenda: Substance abuse/psychosis comorbidity, *Schizophrenia Bulletin*, 33(4): 947-952.

Sass, L. A., and Parnas, J. (2003) Schizophrenia, consciousness and the self, *Schizophrenia Bulletin*, 29(3): 427-444.

Schizophrenia.com (2004) *Negative Symptoms of Schizophrenia,* http://www.schizophrenia.com/diag.ph.

Siegel, A. M. (1996) *Heinz Khout and the Psychology of the Self*, New York: Routledge.

Smith, J., and Hucker, S., (1994) Schizophrenia and substance abuse, *British Journal of Psychiatry* 165: 13-21.

Strauss, G. P., Duke, L. A. Ross, S. A. and Allen, D. N. (2010). Post-traumatic stress disorder and negative symptoms of schizophrenia. *Schizophrenia Bulletin*, 37(3): 1093-1123.

Tart, Charles T. (1969). *Altered States of Consciousness: A Book of Readings*. New York: Wiley.

Thorberg, F. A., and Lyvers, M. T. (2006). Attachment, fear of intimacy and differentiation of *self among clients in substance disorder treatment facilities, Addictive Behaviors, 31: 732–73.*

Ulman, R. B. and Paul, H. (2006). *The Self Psychology of Addiction and Its Treatment: Narcissus in Wonderland*, New York: Routledge.

Vaitl, D. (2012). *Veränderte Bewusstseinszustände: Grundlagen - Techniken - Phänomenologie. Schattauer. p. 14.*

Vollenweider, F. X., and Geyer, M. A. (2001). A system model of altered consciousness: Integrating natural and drug induced psychoses, *Brain Research Bulletin,* 56(5): 495-507.

Williams, L., (2007). *Within Ice Age: A Journal into Crystal-Meth Addiction*, http://www.news.com.au/lifestyle/health/mind/into-the-vortex-luke-williams-spiral-into-iceinduced-psychosis/news-story/73ed84e6830e6192d9685b1de61ed128.

Wurmser, Leon. (1978) *The Hidden Dimension: Psychodynamics in Compulsive Drug Use.* New York : J. Aronson, 1978.

Yip, K. S. (2013) *Emotionality and Mental Illness Vol. 2.* New York: Nova Science Publishers.

Yip, K. S. (2014) *Self-Fragmentation and Self-Integration in People with Schizophrenia, Volume 1: A Multi-dimensional Interpretation and Recovery.* New York: Nova Science Publishers.

Yip, K.S. (2015) *Integrated Dynamic Recovery for People with Substance Abuse and Drug Addiction*. New York: Nova Science Publishers

AUTHOR CONTACT INFORMATION

Kam-shing Yip
Professor
Department of Applied Social Studies,
Hong Kong Polytechnic University,
Hung Hom, Kowloon, Hong Kong
Email: kam-shing.yip@connect.polyu.hk

INDEX

R

S

T

W